# Medicine, Medical Ethics and the Value of Life

### Edited by Peter Byrne

JOHN WILEY & SONS

Chichester · New York · Brisbane · Toronto · Singapore

Copyright © 1990 by John Wiley & Sons Ltd.
Baffins Lane, Chichester
West Sussex PO19 1UD, England

This volume is a continuation of the King's College Studies series of
volumes previously published by King Edward's Hospital Fund for
London.

Distributed in the United States of America, Canada and
Japan by Alan R. Liss Inc., 41 East 11th Street, New York,
NY 10003, USA.

*Other Wiley Editorial Offices*

John Wiley & Sons, Inc., 605 Third Avenue,
New York, NY 10158–0012, USA

Jacaranda Wiley Ltd, G.P.O. Box 859, Brisbane,
Queensland 4001, Australia

John Wiley & Sons (Canada) Ltd, 22 Worcester Road,
Rexdale, Ontario M9W 1L1, Canada

John Wiley & Sons (SEA) Pte Ltd, 37 Jalan Pemimpin 05–04,
Block B, Union Industrial Building, Singapore 2057

**Library of Congress Cataloging-in-Publication Data**

Medicine, medical ethics, and the value of life / edited by Peter
    Byrne.
        p.     cm.
    Includes bibliographical references.
    ISBN 0 471 92516 0
    1. Medical ethics.   2. Life and death, Power over.     I. Byrne,
Peter, 1950–
    [DNLM:   1. Ethics, Medical.     W 50 M4899]
R724.M314   1990
174'.24—dc20
DNLM/DLC
for Library of Congress                                    89–16764
                                                              CIP


**British Library Cataloguing in Publication Data**

Medicine, medical ethics and the value of life.
    1. Medicine. Ethical aspects
    I. Byrne, Peter, 1950–
    174'.2

ISBN 0 471 92516 0

*Parry 17'58 /13·50 11·90*

Typeset by J&L Composition Ltd, Filey, North Yorkshire
Printed and bound in Great Britain by Biddles Ltd., Guildford

This book is due for return on or before the last date shown below.

London, N.21   Cat. No. 1208

# Medicine, Medical Ethics
## and the Value of Life

# Contents

Contributors  vii

Preface  ix
 Peter Byrne

Euthanasia in the Netherlands  1
 H J J Leenen

The BMA on euthanasia: the philosopher
versus the doctor  15
 Peter Byrne

The value of human life  34
 Basil Mitchell

Abortion, embryo research and fetal
transplantation: their moral interrelationships  47
 Sophie Botros

Can medical ethics be taught?  80
 Roger Higgs

Teaching medical ethics: impressions from the USA  89
 Raanan Gillon

The allocation of scarce medical resources:
a democrat's dilemma  116
 Albert Weale

AIDS and tolerance  131
 Richard Harries

The ethics of sex selection  141
 John Mahoney

Index  159

# Contributors

Peter Byrne is a Lecturer in the Philosophy of Religion and a Director of the Centre of Medical Law and Ethics, King's College London.

H J J Leenen is Professor of Social Medicine and Health Law, Academic Medical Centre, University of Amsterdam.

Basil Mitchell was formerly Professor of the Philosophy of Religion in the University of Oxford.

Sophie Botros is a Lecturer in Medical Ethics, King's College London.

Raanan Gillon is Director of the Health Service at Imperial College London, Editor of the *Journal of Medical Ethics* and a Visiting Professor in the Centre of Medical Law and Ethics, King's College London.

Roger Higgs is Director of General Practice Studies and a Director of the Centre of Medical Law and Ethics, King's College London.

Albert Weale is Professor of Politics in the School of Economic and Social Studies, University of East Anglia.

Richard Harries is Bishop of Oxford.

John Mahoney is Professor of Moral and Social Theology and a Director of the Centre of Medical Law and Ethics, King's College London.

# Preface

This volume of King's College studies covers a wide range of issues while focusing on a series of related themes. One group of chapters introduces the question of euthanasia and the value of human life. Professor Leenen's excellent summary of contemporary Dutch legal and ethical thinking on killing in medical practice is juxtaposed with a survey of the British Medical Association's recent report on the law and ethics that govern the duty not to kill in British medical practice. The underlying philosophical opinions on the value of human life and the nature of the harm to be found in killing another person are treated in Basil Mitchell's chapter. The question of what might justify taking human life is also of central importance to Sophie Botros whose chapter ties up some of the loose ends that arise from the discussion of abortion, embryo research and related matters in earlier volumes in this series. Of particular value is her attempt to pin down the sense in one popular way of fixing the worth of human life: that human life is to be treated always as an end and never as a means only. Readers will find her discussion challenging but worth the effort involved in determining the real argumentative force behind this readily used moral tag.

The nature of medical ethics as a discipline, its relationship to clinical practice and to academic study of moral thought is the concern of the chapters contributed by Roger Higgs and Raanan Gillon. One of the important issues emerging from their discussion relates to the help or hindrance that medical ethics, arising from and tested in clinical practice, might receive from academic moralising. Academic moralising is the business of moral philosophers (and moral theologians) and everyone seems to assume that it will be of some help to the real life business of the reflective practice of medicine. The BMA document on euthanasia illustrates the problems that Higgs and Gillon point to in making theory relevant to practice. I also discuss this problem in my own chapter on the BMA report. The BMA working party's refusal to credit the main, agreed point in recent philosophical discussion of the ethics of killing in medicine provides a link between the two groups of chapters described so far. From where and from whom is an ethics of homicide for medicine to come from? How could any such ethics command the assent of society, doctors and academic moralists? These questions are not finally answered in this volume but materials for an answer are assembled, which might be developed in subsequent volumes.

The ethics and policy of the allocation of medical resources and of the treatment and prevention problem of AIDS have been discussed in previous volumes, and these subjects are taken further in the chapters by Albert Weale and Richard Harries. The latter's contribution will prove particularly insightful in appealing to a religious basis for the greatest possible tolerance to AIDS sufferers and HIV-infected individuals. Too often the name and doctrines of established religious traditions are invoked by the unthinking as grounds for making moral examples out of AIDS victims. The Bishop of Oxford shows us exactly what is wrong with this standpoint.

The unthinking also tend to reject the notion that future advances in reproductive medicine should be allowed to grant parents the means of choosing the sex of their offspring. The final chapter challenges us all to consider what, if anything, may be wrong with so extending the power of parents over the future shape of their children's lives. Here John Mahoney's paper will be seen to hinge on a point of consistency. Since we allow medicine proper licence in its ability to mould nature and fight its perceived defects, and since we allow parents considerable liberty in moulding their offsprings' characters, interests, ambitions and the like, what moral and social considerations prevent us limiting reproductive medicine's assistance to parents in the matter of sex selection?

I venture to suggest that this fourth volume of King's College Studies will be found to meet the definition and high standards of worthwhile 'critical medical ethics' set out in Raanan Gillon's contribution.

Peter Byrne

# Euthanasia in the Netherlands

## H J J Leenen

On 11 December 1987, the Dutch government, consisting of Conservatives and Christian Democrats, introduced a draft bill relating to the termination of the life of a patient by a doctor at the patient's express and serious request. The introduction of this proposed law marked a new step in the development of the debate on euthanasia in the Netherlands.[1] This debate started at the beginning of the seventies after the Leeuwarden Court in 1973 stated in its decision on a case that euthanasia would be acceptable if: the patient is incurably ill, the patient suffers unbearably, the patient has requested the termination of his life, and the termination of the patient's life is performed by a doctor who treats the patient or who is being consulted by him.

In the penal code of the Netherlands, euthanasia (section 293) and assistance to suicide (section 294) are prohibited. These sections were included in the penal code in 1891; since then, major changes have occurred in medicine and society. One of the negative concomitants of the progress of medicine is the prolongation of suffering and the disfigurement of dying. Many people consider these effects quite unacceptable and they may request that their life be terminated when the disadvantages of medical treatment outweigh its benefits. In society, norms and values have also changed. The concept of self-determination has become accepted by large parts of the population. People want to take their destiny in their own hands and this wish may manifest itself when, at the end of their life, their situation becomes hopeless and untenable.

Of course opinions differ. Inquiries in the Netherlands

show that an increasing percentage of the population is in favour of (active) euthanasia:

| 1966 | 39.9 per cent |
|------|---------------|
| 1975 | 52.6 per cent |
| 1979 | 51.4 per cent |
| 1980 | 52.4 per cent |
| 1981 | 53.8 per cent |
| 1985 | 67 per cent |
| 1986 | 67 per cent |

In the same period the number of opponents decreased from 48.6 per cent to 17 per cent and, in 1985, as many as 69 per cent of Roman Catholics approved of euthanasia.

Although in the Netherlands the minority is against euthanasia, that opinion has to be respected. In a pluriform society the legislator must aim at legislation which allows for different convictions. If legislation did not prohibit euthanasia, everybody could follow his own conviction. People for and against could live according to their view, thus giving freedom and self-determination to all. Opponents of euthanasia would never expect the legislator to interfere with their freedom: by advocating that their view on euthanasia should be laid down in the law they appear to be inconsistent because they then deny others what they demand for themselves. Apart from that, it shows intolerance of other opinions. It should be added that human self-determination is not derived from the state. Self-determination is an inherent human right. The question is not whether the state must allow for euthanasia but whether the state has reasons to limit human self-determination as to the termination of one's life. This will be discussed later on.

## 1. What euthanasia is and what it is not

It is very important to define precisely what euthanasia is and what it is not. During the debate in the Netherlands, a definition of euthanasia has been developed on which both its advocates and its opponents agree. It can be defined as the deliberate termination of the life of a person at his request by another. Central to this definition is the request of the patient. Without such a request the termination of a life would become murder. It should be emphasised that neither the family, nor other relatives, nor parents for their children, nor the doctor, can decide on behalf of the patient. People who have become incompetent are not thereby more eligible for euthanasia, unless prior to their becoming incompetent they have made a written will in which they ask for the termination of their life. Such a will is only valid when the patient is no longer competent to make up his mind. In all other cases the oral expression of the patient's wishes prevails over the written will.

According to the generally accepted notion of euthanasia the following situations do not fall under the definition of euthanasia. This is also laid down in the law proposal of 11 December 1987.

*a. Not initiating or terminating a medical treatment in cases where such treatment is medically pointless*

Medical treatment is justified by its benefits. Nobody is legally bound to perform pointless acts. When medicine has nothing more to offer, the doctor is not obliged to start or to continue medical treatment. This is also the case when medical treatment is disproportionate to its possible benefits. This judgment can only be made on the basis of medical considerations; non-medical criteria or judgments about the sense or the quality of a patient's life should not play a role. Not initiating or terminating a pointless medical treatment on the basis of purely medical considerations[2] resulting in the death of the patient is not euthanasia. Of course, normal care and sedation of pain should be provided until death.

*b. Painkilling*

The aim of painkilling is to alleviate the patient's suffering, even if this would hasten his death. This shortening of his life is a side-effect. Acts must not be defined according to their side-effects but according to their aims, which is here to alleviate the patient's pain.

*c. Refusal of medical treatment by the patient*

No patient may be treated without his consent and it is his right to refuse treatment or to withdraw his consent. This can result in the death of the patient. Yet the doctor is not allowed to treat in such a case; neither is he liable for the death of the patient. In this context the distinction between active and passive euthanasia has to be discussed. According to the accepted definitions, passive euthanasia would involve abstaining from treatment upon the patient's request. But this is the same as the patient expressing his will not to be treated. So the notion 'passive euthanasia' makes no sense[3] and is best abandoned. It is even hazardous because it would suggest that the termination of the life of a patient by omitting to treat in other than medically pointless cases would be acceptable without his request. Moreover, there is no difference between acting and omitting when acting is a duty. Again the distinction between active and passive euthanasia makes no sense.

## 2. The role of the courts

After the decision of the Leeuwarden Court in 1973, mentioned before, the Dutch courts have judged in several other cases: the Court of Rotterdam (1981); the Court of Alkmaar (1983) with appeal to the Court of Appeals of Amsterdam (1983); a decision of the Supreme Court (1984) and referral to the Court of Appeals of The Hague (1986); the Court of Groningen (1984) with appeal to the Court of Appeals of Leeuwarden (1984); a decision of the Supreme Court (1986) and referral to the Court of Appeals of Arnhem (1987); the Court of Rotterdam (1985) with appeal to the Court of Appeals of The Hague (1987); the Court of The Hague (1985); the Court of The Hague (1985) with appeal to the Court of Appeals of The Hague (1986) followed by a decision of the Disciplinary Court of The Hague (1987); the Court of Appeals of Arnhem (1986) brought before the Supreme Court (1987); the Court of Almelo (1988). The Disciplinary Court of Amsterdam judged a case in 1977 and again in 1985 with appeal to the Central Disciplinary Court (1986). The same case was also judged by the Court of Haarlem (1986). All these decisions concern doctors. In their rulings the courts set criteria and standards to be followed by the doctor when administering euthanasia. In two cases, nurses and a nursing assistant (Court of Amsterdam 1988, Court of Rotterdam 1987) were involved. Disregarding other aspects of these decisions (assistant) nurses were not allowed to decide on euthanasia.

Space does not permit discussion of all these separate

decisions.[4] I will therefore limit myself to the ruling of the Supreme Court which sets standards for the lower courts on the legal possibilities of acquittal of a doctor under the existing penal code which prohibits euthanasia. The lawyers defending the doctors advocated the following arguments when pleading for the acquittal of their clients.

a. Euthanasia does not fall under sections 293 and 294 of the penal code because the legislator did not intend to include the termination of the life of a suffering patient in the said criminal acts. This argument, which did not find much support in literature, was rejected by the Supreme Court.

b. Euthanasia is not materially wrong because although it comes formally under the wording of the said sections, it is justified. In this argument a comparison was drawn with normal medical acts, such as surgery, which come under the criminal law but are justified. The Supreme Court rejected this way of reasoning.

c. Euthanasia is normal medical practice and thus does not fall under the penal code. This argument also met with disapproval. Here the Supreme Court followed the distinction made in health law between medical acts according to the medical professional standard and acts which, although they are mostly carried out by doctors, are governed by social rules. Abortion and euthanasia, *sub alia*, are of the latter category. It is not up to the medical profession to set rules allowing abortion and euthanasia. This is a matter for society to decide and not for the medical profession.

d. *Force majeure*, in the sense of conflicting duties, allows for euthanasia. In the Dutch penal code, *force majeure* can create an exception and the Supreme Court accepted in all its decisions that euthanasia was an exception. In the wording of the first ruling the Supreme Court decided that the Court of Appeals did not investigate 'whether according to responsible medical judgment, tested by norms of medical ethics, *force majeure* existed in this case'. In this case the Court of Appeals could, for instance, have attached importance to: whether and, if so, to what extent, according to professional medical judgment, increasing deterioration of the patient's personality and/or increasing deterioration of his already unbearable

suffering were to be expected; whether, also taking into
account the possibility of new serious relapses, it was to be
expected that soon he would no longer be in the position to die
with dignity; whether and, if so, to what extent there were
other ways of alleviating his suffering.[5] Because the Court of
Appeals of Amsterdam had not considered these factors, the
Supreme Court reversed its decision and referred the case to
the Court of Appeals of The Hague which acquitted the
doctor. Although the Supreme Court can not ignore the law, it
nevertheless made an opening for acquittal of doctors administering euthanasia under certain conditions. Because the courts
are bound by the law, the need for new legislation remains.

## 3. Proposals for legislation

Several arguments exist for legislation on euthanasia. First it
has to be absolutely certain that the termination of the life of a
patient will only be administered on request of the patient.
There must be no doubt that the termination of his life is his
explicit and serious wish. The legislator has to see that such a
decision of the patient is made freely and without the influence
of third parties. Protection of self-determination is one of the
duties of the legislator. Second, euthanasia is administered by
another person, namely the doctor. In general, legal protection
must be guaranteed when third parties make decisions for
people; the more so when such decisions involve the termination of the life of a patient. Doctors are emotionally very much
involved with a patient for whom the end of life is in sight and it
must be guaranteed that the said decision is made very
carefully. Other arguments are that in a democratic society it is
up to parliament to set the rules for euthanasia and that
legislation is required to guarantee that every case is treated
equally. Moreover, practical experience suggests that without
legislation it is not clear on which criteria the prosecution may
decide to bring a case before the court and the criteria applied
by the courts depend on the facts of the case and diverge
accordingly. This causes a problem for the doctor because he
has to make up his mind *ex ante* and the courts rule *ex post*
judging whether, in his case, the doctor was right to invoke
*force majeure*.

In 1982 the government took two decisions. First it decided

that all decisions as to future prosecutions should be discussed in a joint meeting of the heads of the prosecution service on the basis of existing court rulings (by then Leeuwarden 1973 and Rotterdam 1981). However, the decisions of those controlling the prosecution service are not public. Another problem is that by this procedure the prosecution adopts the role of 'pseudo legislator'. The second step was to establish a State Commission on Euthanasia. In the Dutch system a State Commission is the highest ranked type of committee; it is appointed by the Queen. The State Commission consisted of 15 members drawn from different professional and religious backgrounds. The Commission reported in August 1985 and the report was adopted by 13 votes to 2. In the meantime, one of the political parties in parliament took the initiative to submit a draft law to parliament. The other political parties, however, were not inclined to follow this initiative, preferring to wait for the report of the State Commission.

The report discussed many issues – for example, minors, incompetent adults, prisoners, conscious objections, the role of nurses, pharmacists and the like. Central to the report was a proposal for a law. The following focuses upon this proposal.[6]

The nucleus is an amendment of the penal code. The State Commission was in favour of maintaining the existing rule that a person who intentionally terminates the life of another person on his explicit and serious request is punishable. But it proposed to add a second paragraph stating that this act is not punishable when the termination of the life is administered by a physician, within the framework of careful medical practice, to a patient who is in an untenable situation without any prospects. In the explanatory note it is argued that further delineation of this criterion is not possible because every individual situation is different. In a third paragraph, assistance to suicide, in as far as it complies with the criteria for euthanasia, is put on a par with euthanasia.

In the fourth paragraph the minimum requirements for careful medical practice are elaborated. These requirements are that:

a. the patient has to be informed about his situation;

b. the physician must have become convinced that the patient's request for the termination of his life is the result of careful consideration and that he has upheld his request freely;

c. the physician must judge that the termination of the patient's life is justified, because on the basis of his findings together with the patient he has come to the conclusion that there is no alternative to the untenable situation of the patient;

d. the physician has to consult another physician.

These criteria and the criteria developed by the courts are essentially the same.

The fifth paragraph deals with the written request.

After publication of the State Commission's report the draft of the proposed law was adapted to the report. The government and the Christian Democrats who were in office, were unwilling to adhere to the draft which was supported by a majority in parliament. Therefore the government took the unusual step of publishing a draft of a Bill of its own without giving it the formal status of a proposed law. The government said that should parliament proceed with the pending draft, it would formally introduce its own proposal. In March 1986 the debate in parliament took place. In this debate the Conservative Party withdrew its support for the proposed law because of the problems likely to arise within the government in which the Conservatives were represented: they would not risk the fall of the government. The result of the parliamentary debate was that both proposals were submitted to the State Council.

In the meantime the public debate went on. In May 1986, elections for parliament were held. As a result, the Conservatives and the Christian Democrats continued their coalition. During the formation of the cabinet both parties agreed that the opinion of the State Council was to be abided by and a decision-making procedure was agreed upon. A few days after this agreement the opinion of the State Council was published. The Council, forced into the uncomfortable position of an arbitrator, came up with a rather ambivalent opinion. Although the State Council advised postponing legislation, the government could not adopt a position of wait and see, because the public debate was still going on and the 1984 proposed law was still pending in parliament. So both parties in government worked on a compromise which was published on 16 January 1987 and which led to the draft of a law on 11 December 1987. By introducing a draft of a law, the government deviated from the opinion of the State Council.

The nucleus of the compromise is that the physician administering euthanasia will remain punishable. The State Commission on Euthanasia and the proposal pending in parliament are of the opinion that a physician administering euthanasia according to the rules would not be punishable. However, in the government's draft a new section is to be included in the Medical Practice Act outlining the requirements for careful medical practice when performing euthanasia. These requirements essentially follow the proposal of the State Commission on Euthanasia, with addition of the rules that the physician has to find out whether the patient is prepared to involve his close relatives in the decision on euthanasia and that the physician – provided the patient does not object to this – has to consult the close relatives on whether the request of the patient has been freely made, and maintained, after careful consideration. (There are several arguments against pressing the patient to involve close relatives. For instance, the privacy of the patient may be threatened. Furthermore, close relatives are often not able to make objective judgments because of their personal involvement, or the effect of the patient's illness on their own lives, or because they may start a mourning process when the patient is still alive which may influence their opinion, or because of a possible interest in the inheritance.) The next requirement is that the physician has to make a report. But apart from these additions, the main problem of the government draft is that the doctor, even when he has followed the requirements to be laid down in the Medical Practice Act, remains punishable and can only invoke *force majeure*, to be assessed by the prosecution and the judge. There is no connection between the rules in the Medical Practice Act and the penal code. In this compromise the Christian Democrats have upheld their position that euthanasia is punishable, while the Conservatives have included in the law the criteria for careful medical practice to be followed by a physician performing euthanasia. As often happens with compromises, the government draft is a half-way step. It disregards the opinion of the majority of the population which is in favour of impunity for a doctor who administers euthanasia according to the rules. In mid-1988 the situation was that the government draft has to go through the preparatory procedures in parliament, after which the two drafts are open for parliamentary debate.

## 4. The euthanasia debate

The main argument of those who approve of euthanasia is based upon human self-determination. They do not approve of a state that is allowed to impose on its citizens ethical rules that interfere with their private lives. For such an encroachment upon individual rights to be valid, strong arguments need to be available to show that without such interfering rules essential values of society would be endangered. This is not the case when patients suffering severely and unbearably at the end of their lives request the termination of their suffering when no alternatives exist. Not allowing people euthanasia would come down to forcing them to suffer against their will, which would be cruel and a negation of their human rights and dignity. Dying in dignity is the last good a human being can experience; and everyone should be allowed this. The progress of modern medicine and technology has greatly influenced the process of dying for the better and for the worse. In some cases the negative effects can become enormous. Should medicine be allowed to manipulate nature in one way but forbidden to obliterate its own negative effects? New developments in medicine and technology have consequences for human self-determination; because they affect the process of dying, human self-determination has been extended to this process of dying. One cannot let science expand freely and disregard the consequences for human responsibility.

For the state this can result in the need for new protective measures in order to guarantee human freedom and self-determination. A classic role for the state is to act as a safeguard of human rights. As to human freedom, the state's position is ambivalent: freedom has to be protected by and against the state. As discussed before, the state must not encroach upon human freedom by imposing ethical rules interfering with the private lives of citizens and, at the same time, its responsibility is to safeguard individual freedom and self-determination. Because decision-making on euthanasia is a subtle process which places a lot of strain on the exercise of human self-determination there are arguments for euthanasia legislation in order to protect this self-determination. These arguments are at the basis of the proposals for legislation, discussed in section 3.

The opponents of euthanasia put forward several kinds of arguments to support their stand. Some are motivated by their religious convictions and these convictions have to be respected. It is within the scope of their self-determination to reject euthanasia. Another argument is that it is a duty of the state to protect life. Indeed, the state has to protect its citizens against their lives being taken against their will. But it is different when it is done at a person's explicit request. By definition individual rights aim at protecting freedom from interference of the state and of third parties; they are not intended to restrict the freedom of the individual. The individual himself can dispose of his life and in many cases this is not only accepted but praised – for instance, when one sacrifices one's life to save another person's life. In many countries suicide is not illegal. The state has to ensure that everyone is free to make decisions about his own life. As a consequence, euthanasia which by definition is upon request of the person concerned, does not fall under article 2 of the European Convention for the Protection of Human Rights and Fundamental Freedoms (1950). This article states that everyone's life will be protected by law and that no one will be deprived of his life, save in explicitly described cases. It prohibits the state and others from taking someone's life against his will, but provides no basis for the prohibition of the termination of a person's life at his own free will.

The opponents of euthanasia often use the 'slippery slope' argument: allowing euthanasia, which by definition is on request, will eventually result in the termination of life without request. This objection is unconvincing. To make it acceptable it has to be demonstrated that the consequences which are feared will eventually occur; that they are caused by the social acceptance of euthanasia and not by other factors; that the said consequences cannot be prevented; and that they will not occur when euthanasia is prohibited by law. Experience shows that the slippery slope argument is weak. The argument, for instance, was also used in the abortion debate; however, after the adoption of the Abortion Law in the Netherlands there was no increase in the number of abortions. Equally, with euthanasia, a slippery slope is not to be expected. Unrequested termination of life would encroach

upon the rights of grandparents, parents and, in the end, everybody.[7]
Referring to involuntary termination of lives under the Nazi regime is a false argument. That the Nazis used the term euthanasia for murder constitutes no case against euthanasia. Murder of innocent victims on the basis of an obscene fascist philosophy may not be compared with helping people to terminate their unbearable suffering at their own request in a democratic constitutional state based upon human rights. Recognising and respecting individual rights is totally different from trampling people's rights underfoot.

Some doubt whether a patient is able to make a decision about the termination of his life. However, denying patients the competency to do so would essentially result in putting aside patients' rights. Moreover, everybody accepts that patients have to consent to medical treatment and that it is their right to refuse treatment, even when this would lead to death. Why, then, should they not be able to make up their minds on euthanasia? Furthermore, experience shows that many terminally ill patients are very lucid, have intense contacts with their relatives and are capable of arranging their affairs. It would be an injustice to the dying to declare them incompetent. This does not alter the fact that for euthanasia the free request of the patient is vital; this condition is laid down in the Dutch law proposals and is strongly ruled in all Dutch court decisions. Here written requests also play a role. To assess the patient's wish, a good relationship between the doctor and the patient is of great importance.

Another argument by opponents is that making euthanasia permissible would undermine the trust of the public in health care and of patients in their doctors. This will not happen, as experience shows, when patients can be convinced that without their explicit request no euthanasia will take place. On the contrary, because everybody knows that the termination of life has always been part of medical practice, even when euthanasia was not permitted by law, patients often feel insecure in this respect. Legalising euthanasia gives patients a feeling of protection that their lives will not be terminated without their explicit request. Moreover, many patients appreciate that they can discuss euthanasia freely with their doctors and this decreases their anxiety that their life has to end with unbearable suffering. Often, when a doctor has promised the patient that he will help him when the situation has become untenable, the patient relaxes and the wish to receive euthanasia is postponed. Bringing euthanasia into the open has a positive effect on patients and on their relationships with doctors.

Opponents also argue that allowing euthanasia will undermine doctors' morale. But everybody who knows how much strain administering euthanasia puts upon the doctor, even when he is convinced that euthanasia is the only option, will not accept this argument. On the contrary, doctors often feel demoralised by the knowledge that euthanasia is punishable and that the law does not allow them to help their severely suffering patients. This does not imply that control mechanisms to safeguard careful decision-making do not have to be established.

Finally, there are arguments relating to the uncertainty of medicine. The diagnosis may be wrong, new therapies may become available and miracles may happen. These arguments are unconvincing. The possibility of a wrong diagnosis is always present in medicine. Nevertheless, doctors do not refrain from administering medicine. In the case of cessation of a medically pointless treatment a wrong diagnosis can occur, but this will not prevent doctors from terminating such treatment. But, more important, euthanasia may only be administered to a severely ill patient whose illness has reached a final stage. Then there is no doubt that the patient is incurably ill. The chance that a new therapy will be discovered out of the blue is negligible. Unless there are indications to the contrary in the medico-scientific community, it is unreasonable to expect new therapies to become available that quickly. The same is true for miracles! Human behaviour cannot be guided by the possibility of miracles. It would be inhuman to deny the patient an end to his suffering with an appeal to a miracle which is improbable and not to be expected.

## 5. Conclusion

Euthanasia is a universal and long-standing problem which has often been shrouded in secrecy. In the Netherlands, however, it has been openly debated since 1973 and it has only been possible, within the limits of this chapter, to discuss the main points of the debate and to outline the main proposals for legislation. It is not yet clear, though, exactly what kind of legislation will result from the wish to lay down rules for euthanasia in the law.

## Notes and references

1. In the Netherlands, no difference is made between euthanasia and assistance to suicide when given under the same circumstances as euthanasia. For this reason only the term euthanasia will be used.

2. The guidelines on the termination of life-sustaining treatment and the care of the dying (New York, Hastings Center, 1987) say: if a treatment is clearly futile, in the sense that it will not achieve its physiological objective and so bring no physiological benefits to the patient, there is no obligation to provide the treatment.

3. Sometimes not initiating or terminating a medically pointless treatment is called passive euthanasia. This is incorrect because it is not euthanasia.

4. Elements of the court rules are discussed in H J J Leenen. Euthanasia, assistance to suicide and the law: developments in the Netherlands. Health Policy, 8, 2, 1987, pages 197–206. For the first decision of the Supreme Court see H J J Leenen. Supreme Court's decision on euthanasia in the Netherlands. Medicine and Law, 5, 1986, pages 349–351.

5. The Supreme Court's decision was approved by the greater part of the scientific and lay press. It was only criticised because it referred to medical ethics.

6. See Final report of the Netherlands State Commission on Euthanasia: an English summary. Bioethics, 2, April 1987, pages 163–174.

7. J Weinfeld. Active voluntary euthanasia: should it be legalized? Medicine and Law, 4, 1985, pages 101–111.

# The BMA on euthanasia: the philosopher versus the doctor

Peter Byrne

The BMA's report on euthanasia[1] inevitably invites comparison with the excellent account and defence of current practice in the Netherlands offered by Professor Leenen in the previous chapter. Indeed it takes the trouble to comment on the licence given to euthanasia by social policy in the Netherlands, and presents a sharp contrast between practice and policy in the UK and practice and policy there. The BMA document also raises at least one other main point of interest to readers of this volume. In his paper on the teaching of medical ethics, Dr Raanan Gillon defends the importance of what he styles 'critical medical ethics' to the practice of medicine. It is clear, both from his presentation of the matter and from the character of the literature published, that critical medical ethics depends to a large extent on the use of moral philosophy and moral philosophers to provide a commentary on the issues raised by clinical practice. This volume contains chapters by Sophie Botros and Basil Mitchell which continue the contemporary attempt to use philosophical analysis to illuminate and mould medical practice. Put simply, the BMA report raises the question of whether this attempt is at all worthwhile. Its content fuels doubts about whether philosophers and reflective medical practitioners can communicate successfully. How it brings these issues to the fore is best discussed after the differences between UK and Dutch practice with regard to euthanasia are set out.

The chief reasons why the BMA working party was able to reject the Dutch model for an ethics of euthanasia boil down to two: a question of fact and question of the purpose and function of law.

The persistent argument of the BMA report (see especially chapters 2 and 10) is that the kind of circumstances which Professor Leenen describes as presenting the doctor with the moral necessity of killing in order to relieve suffering need not arise, and do not arise, in this country. Techniques for the management of pain and terminal illness, as pioneered by the hospice movement, mean that few patients ever reach the stage where they have a persistent wish to be killed and the doctor feels that the only thing he can do for them is to accede to that request. The report indeed implies that it is because the development of palliative care is not so well advanced in the Netherlands that the advocacy of euthanasia is taken so seriously in that country.

As a medical layman I can offer little intelligent comment on this side of the BMA's case. The chief difficulty, described below, relates to its inconsistency. This inconsistency weakens the contrast drawn between British medical practice which, the BMA affirms, will not kill in order to save from suffering, and Dutch practice which will.

Professor Leenen's case for the legalisation of medical killing in appropriate circumstances depends in large measure on the argument that the function of law is to promote the autonomy of individuals, provided their exercise of that autonomy does not harm others. The BMA makes much of the fact (and is surely right in doing so) that the function of statute and common law in this country cannot be seen in those terms. The facts that aiding and abetting a suicide is a statutory crime and that consent of the victim is not a defence against a charge of murder indicate the weight behind this view. While it appears that the law will allow some harms to the person to escape criminality if consented to, 'There are limits to the right of any person to consent to the infliction of physical harm on himself'.[2]

If we accept that this is law and social policy as it now stands then there are two main issues to be considered in deciding whether it needs modifying.

Should bringing about a human being's death be regarded as a grievous harm in all circumstances? The groundwork for answering this vital (philosophical?) question is admirably laid in Professor Mitchell's chapter, where the main, contending schools of thought are described. I shall offer no further comment on it immediately, but will later raise once again the question of how far the BMA is consistent in its approach to this and other issues it treats.

Should not the law change so as to adopt the stance of seeking to promote individual autonomy to the maximum degree? The defence of voluntary euthanasia fits in well with a liberal philosophy of the function of law which holds that it should serve only to prevent individuals from harming one another or from pursuing conduct which interferes with the freedom of others to follow their plans of life. Law and social regulation should offer the minimum constraints necessary to promote the maximum liberty of all. This philosophy is in fundamental conflict with much of the content of law and social regulation in this country (as shown in the discussion of AIDS, public health and liberty in King's College Studies for 1987–8).[3,4] Much legislation is concerned with protecting individuals from harms deemed too serious to place within the liberty of the subject (consider, for example, our drugs legislation). This is indeed one of the weaknesses of basing a case for voluntary euthanasia on a duty of legislators to maximise individual liberty wherever possible. Recognition of that duty would involve major and far-ranging changes in law. Moreover, it appears odd to begin an attempt to make social regulation conform to this ideal by concentrating on establishing a liberty or right to choose the time and manner of death while under medical care. The limits on individual autonomy presented by restrictions on euthanasia appear to be minor, incidental aspects of what some see as authoritarian and paternalistic aspects of social policy at present. A large scale crusade would have to be launched to achieve Professor Leenen's ideal. Why begin it here?

It might be argued that we have good reason to begin a crusade for the advancement of autonomy through focusing on an issue in medical practice. The requirement of the informed consent of patients already embodies an existing ideal of maximising autonomy and this only needs to be extended to 'the right to die'. Much has been made of the move within contemporary doctrine of informed consent away from the merely negative concern with defences against battery and negligence towards a recognition of patient autonomy as an ideal.[5] However, in the common law tradition consent is not a sufficient condition for a licit medical intervention on the person or in the life of a patient. There must in addition be a reasonable degree of skill in performing the intervention and an expectation of benefit to the patient from the intervention.[6] (Where non-therapeutic, research procedures are undertaken this last condition requires that no substantial harm stems from the procedures.) So the question remains of whether an intervention designed to kill a patient can be construed as anything other than one which brings harm to him. Where consent and autonomy are made much of in medical ethics they are most plausible if seen as encapsulating factors which make a genuine partnership or moral relationship possible between doctor and patient. But then they cannot be regarded as licences to demand of the doctor procedures which bypass his own conscientious judgment as to what is harmful or not to human beings. They are conditions which prevent the doctor–patient relationship being manipulative of the patient, not ones which enable the relationship to become manipulative of the doctor.

The fact that common law and much reflective ethical opinion bids a doctor to respect a firm decision on behalf of the patient to refuse life-saving treatment and thus, in effect, choose death cannot be used to overturn these points about consent and the limits of autonomy. The requirements in the common law tradition for licit medical treatment lay at least two duties on the doctor, the violation of either of which makes medical practice improper: not to treat without explicit or tacit consent and not to treat without a reasonable expectation of benefit (or a reasonable expectation that no harm will come to a patient). Forced treatment to save life against the patient's declared and certain wishes violates the first of these duties. If we regard killing as always a form of harm, as social policy *appears* to do at present, then effecting even voluntary euthanasia is contrary to the second of these duties.

The main problem with these defences of existing medical and legal opinion on euthanasia in the UK is also the one that raises the question of whether doctors and philosophers can profitably communicate in medical ethics. The opinion that killing patients is harming them and that there are no circumstances, short of treatment on the battlefield or in cataclysmic disasters, in which doctors need to bring about death as the means of saving their patients from suffering and indignity, is only plausible to the extent that existing ways of managing the dying, the handicapped new-born and the senile can be distinguished from seeking to kill in order to ward off evil. We all know, and the BMA report acknowledges the fact in some detail, that in many approved and accepted medical procedures the hastening of death, to put it no stronger, is the foreseen outcome of the doctor's acts or omissions. The possibility arises of a massive inconsistency between, on the one hand, the propositions that death is not to be pursued as a benefit for patients and that euthanasia is not necessary for sound medicine, and, on the other, the actual state of medical opinion and practice. The main device which the BMA report uses to distance the acceptance of hastened death from the pursuit of death as a goal and benefit in medicine is the distinction between killing and letting die. Doctors are not to kill, have no need of killing in normal circumstances, but they can and do make treatment decisions which have the effect of letting patients die. It so happens that one of the few points which philosophical writers on the ethics of homicide agree upon is that the killing/letting die distinction is not to be relied on in a general form. It masks distinctions which ought to be made clear. Omitting to save or prolong life can often amount, morally speaking, to killing. If this impressive testimony can be dismissed in a major report from a leading medical body, what is the point of analytic moral philosophy as a tool for the alleged illumination of medical practice? In three pages (24–26) the members of the BMA working party, which included only one individual with philosophical training as an 'observer', refuse to credit the many philosophical arguments for distrusting the killing/letting die distinction and simply back the practitioner's hunch that killing and letting die are clearly and essentially different. In contrast, Professor Leenen accepts in his chapter that the distinction between active and passive euthanasia is misleading and mischievous.

I shall indicate below some major points of controversy over the comparative morality of acts and omissions within contemporary philosophical debate, but there is widespread agreement on at least the following: that it is possible through an act of omission to enact an intention to bring about death; that it is therefore possible to kill through omission; that decisions not to treat made by doctors can amount to killing patients if death is one of the foreseen and intended results of the omission of life-saving treatment. If these assertions are indeed correct, then any general use of the killing/letting die distinction will lead to confusion and obfuscation, since there are likely to be some killings through non-treatment and inaction which hide under the label 'letting die'. The philosophical claims about killing through omission can rest on a variety of grounds, some of them highly theoretical and abstract. But there is considerable common sense behind the view that a doctor has killed his patient through omission, or at least hastened his death, if he has the opportunity to save or prolong that patient's life through some available treatment but deliberately withholds that treatment in the knowledge that death will occur or be hastened as a result of withholding it, and does so with the purpose that death should occur. The law is no stranger to the idea that one can kill through omission. Parents who succeed in killing unwanted infants through deliberate starvation are guilty of murder. Given opportunity, knowledge and intent, it appears obvious that an agent may be equally responsible for the results of his refrainings as for those which follow from his positive actions, and that with these conditions (opportunity, knowledge, intent) and the right surrounding circumstances killing may be performed by refraining. So in many circumstances, to let someone die when the means and opportunity exist to save him is to kill him. 'Letting die' is often a euphemism for 'killing'.

Philosophers of a consequentialist persuasion will add to these considerations the claim, central to their theoretical undertaking in moral philosophy, that there is no difference in general between the morality of acts and omissions. They hold that we are equally responsible for the consequences of our refrainings as for our positive actions in all circumstances where we can foresee such consequences. Other philosophers object that this view entails an impossible rigorism in morality which would reduce our respect for special moral prohibitions. For example, it entails that I am responsible for the deaths of the starving in Africa which have occurred while I have been writing this chapter, since I could have devoted my efforts to raising money for them instead of contributing to this book. Non-consequentialist philosophers prefer to argue that some element of positive intent to kill, or real negligence arising out of a failure to live up to special obligations to care for those concerned, is necessary to make an individual morally accountable for another's death (compare Kuhse,[7] Devine[8] and Linacre Centre[9] for different views on the claims of consequentialism about omissions). But it is plain that even if intent and special responsibility are necessary to make the label 'killing' appropriate, it is still possible to kill through omission. We need not embrace a consequentialist moral philosophy to suspect the distinction between killing and letting die. In fact the condition of special responsibility for caring for another is established in the doctor–patient relationship. It is also true that in the types of killing/hastening of death the BMA would like to call 'letting die' the doctor acts foreseeing that death (or the hastening of death) will result from his non-treatment.

It would be extremely neat to be able to argue in all the cases styled 'letting die' that, though the bringing about of death was foreseen as a consequence of non-treatment, it was not actually intended. If this were the case the killing/letting die distinction would be a simple consequence of the distinction between death as one of the purposes of an agent's acts and death as merely the expected side-effect of action (direct versus indirect killing as some writers like to put it[8]). Medical killing through omission would not really be killing if the principle of double effect were then relied on to produce the conclusion that medical letting die occurred when the primary intent behind non-treatment was to avoid the infliction of a burdensome treatment, hastened death being merely a foreseen side-effect. However, it is impossible to argue that this is the case. The terms of the BMA's own discussion of the facts show that many deaths-through-non-treatment cannot be described as indirect killings following this model. Many treatments that are licitly withheld are ones which are in themselves burdensome and they are withheld for the reason that the additional burden they produce should not be inflicted on the patient. The hastened death of the patient is not purposed, planned or striven for, albeit that it is foreseen. Yet when we read pages 35–37 of the BMA document we see that some treatments are burdensome, and therefore withheld, on the very ground that the life they would prolong is burdensome. They are withheld because that life is judged not worth prolonging in its present state and because the doctor is unable to do anything that will significantly improve it. It is the burden of further living that the doctor wishes to prevent and his omission is intended to remove that burden:

> ... for some patients life as a whole is an intolerable burden; they are, despite counselling and support, in pain, distress, incontinent, upset at their insight into the fact that they are severely deformed or disabled, or becoming demented. In such conditions it is not the treatment as such that constitutes cruelty but the medical prolongation of life, by however gentle the means. Where the only outcome of treatment is further suffering then it seems that the right thing to do is to agree not to take any further measures which merely prolong life and cannot relieve suffering (page 35). (Kuhse has the same point[7] and Professor Mitchell presses it in criticism of the Linacre Centre report on euthanasia.[9])

What is this but the frank admission that some forms of non-treatment are intended to bring about death? The grounds for forming and acting upon such an intention are exactly those defenders of open euthanasia would advance: there are circumstances where little can be done to ease a patient's suffering or distress except to bring about or hasten his death. The killing/letting die distinction has no content when used to describe such cases.

The only substantial ground for refusing to describe non-treatment in these instances as a form of killing is offered on page 24 of the BMA document:

> ... action to terminate a patient's life is irrevocable and allows no respite for reevaluation, whereas a decision not to prolong life is often capable of reappraisal once the patient experiences the true implications of the step he has taken.

We might rephrase the point as follows: the doctor in these cases has formed and acted upon only a hesitant and conditional intention to bring about his patient's death. This will still not allow us to see any great difference between positive and negative medical killings, for it is presumably possible in principle to use active, lethal agents which have gradual, reversible results. In any event, if the doctor carries his intent to bring about or hasten the patient's death through to its outcome, it will at some stage have changed its character. The reversible policy will become irreversible.

There is another fact about these deaths through omission that may be alleged to differentiate them from real killings. They are opportunistic. The doctor does not place the patient's life in danger; indeed he does everything possible to avoid that danger. Once it is in peril, however, he may take up the option of non-treatment leading to death if circumstances justify this. Now we might ask: 'Is someone really guilty of killing another if he refuses to save him from a mortal danger for which he is not responsible?' We might imagine that an agent would not be found guilty of murder if he simply refused to save someone from a mortal threat which was not of his own making. If I came across a child drowning in a shallow stream and refused to come to his aid, I might escape a charge of homicide and might be thought to be less guilty, from a moral point of view, than one who actually initiates a process which threatens another's life. But this kind of reflection conceals distinctions once more. One ground which might influence us in regarding the non-life-saver as less morally guilty of another's death is that his omission might not proceed from an intent to kill. Mere indifference or laziness may be all that is behind the omission of life-saving action. Such a person is not a killer because he does not enact an intention to kill through an act of omission. He is instead morally culpable of callousness or shocking indifference to the lives of others. This kind of omission of life-saving means through indifference cannot be at all analogous to 'letting die' in clinical practice. There we are viewing deliberate, thoughtful decisions that some lives are so poor in quality that their continuation is not to be striven for. Moreover, those with the responsibility for caring for one whose life is threatened might well be open to charges of murder or manslaughter if they knowingly or negligently fail to ward off life-threatening evils confronting those in their care. Parents who so acted towards one of their children might be legally and morally guilty of killing him because of the special relationship they had with the victim of their neglect. We can certainly affirm that their intent to let him die would require just as strenuous a justification as a non-opportunistic intent to kill. Could we imagine any circumstances where opportune bringing about of death of this kind was morally justified but more active killing was not? What is true of the duties arising out of the special relationship between parent and child holds equally for those arising out of the doctor–patient relationship, for in that too special obligations are assumed by one entrusted with the care of the potentially weak and vulnerable.

It may be urged in defence of the special nature of medical 'letting die' that in many cases of death arising out of non-treatment the patient's early death was inevitable and the omission of further life-prolonging measures was not really an important cause of death. It merely hastened death somewhat. Here lies a difficult point. It has been said that, since all must die, killing and hastening death are equivalent.[2] Yet it is clear that we would not begin to think of non-treatment as a cause of death if treatment could only have prolonged life by an extra second. We have no criteria for deciding by exactly how much hastening death becomes causing death and killing. It must be pointed out, however, that the option of non-treatment when treatment would only prolong useless life would not be a serious one unless it were the case that the prolongation to be forgone was significant. If the medical prolongation of life that was possible was not significant then it could not be described as a 'cruelty' to be avoided. The exact extent of the causal role of non-treatment in bringing about death is not that morally important if we adopt the stance of the BMA and place great stress on the doctor's intentions in working out the moral character of his acts. What then matters is whether or not he intended a significant help to an early death through omission.

The devices used to distinguish intended death through omission in medicine from full-blown killing may or may not carry conviction. But they cease to be of vital interest once we realise that there is a range of cases of 'letting die' described and accepted as licit in the BMA report which give no scope for their use. I refer particularly to the bringing about of the death of severely handicapped or malformed infants (though the point partly applies also to the practices described by the BMA in relation to adult patients in a persistent vegetative state). The crucial fact that makes 'non-treatment' (itself a euphemism in this context) something which cannot be separated from killing is that the death of many of these infants is sought precisely because it is *not* certain that they are dying. With treatment they could be given at least some chance of a fair span of life. An assessment is made of the infant's likely future handicap or of his likely capacity to respond to and communicate with others. If these assessments are sufficiently gloomy then it is deemed wrong to allow him to live on. Death is then brought about through non-treatment. In some instances, as the BMA notes on page 46, the steps taken to bring death about will be fairly active and include sedation so that the child will not demand sufficient food to live. The BMA working party is careful to note the range of different cases that come in this general category and the differences within medical opinion about exactly how much treatment and help to offer to handicapped infants. Yet two facts remain evident; that there are a significant number of cases where paediatricians arrange for the deaths of handicapped infants on the ground that their future quality of life is too low; and that the BMA respects this practice as within the range of responsible, reasonable medical conduct. This is medical killing on quality of life grounds, and far from it being the case that the active use of lethal agents is incompatible with the intentions behind it, the concern for the suffering and quality of life of infants that motivates it should bid that doctors use such agents as will enable the business of dying (which must in some cases be distressing to both infant and observers alike) to be as swift as possible.[7]

It is appropriate to summarise the points made so far. The BMA has argued that doctors remain legally and morally obligated not to kill and that in normal medical practice there are no circumstances where they need to plead to social morality or law to release them from this duty. In normal circumstances, their duty to care for their patients' well-being does not conflict with their duty not to kill. They have contended that the duty to care and comfort does sometimes absolve them of the duty to prolong life and therefore that they are allowed to let patients die. But the more we examine the category of letting die the more we see that it is not a homogeneous one and that it includes instances of acts which are morally equivalent to killing. So it is the case after all that UK medical practice is shaped by the belief that in some instances the duty not to kill clashes with the duty to care, and that sometimes the duty not to kill should give way before the duty to care. Attention to philosophical reflection could and should have made these points plain, because enough philosophical work has been done to convince the intelligent that the phrase 'letting die' in the description of medical practice covers too many heterogeneous cases to be relied on when discussing the application of the ethics of homicide to this area.

The question remains: Why did the BMA working party feel able to ignore the weight of philosophical commentary on acts and omissions in the ethics of homicide? The answer can best be indicated when we consider what might justify the 'lettings die' in medicine that amount to homicide. I shall concentrate on the bringing about of death in paediatric care to probe this question of what might justify medical acts which to all intents and purposes are homicides. One justification for killing severely handicapped infants might be found in the notion that, prior to the achievement of self-consciousness, *no* human infant is to be counted as a person. They have not yet acquired the capacities that make something a person – for example, the ability to envision their future and to form a self-conscious desire to go on living. Not being selfconscious creatures they are unable to value their own lives and their lives do not then deserve the unique protection we afford to the lives of persons. The wrong in killing young infants is largely the harm it does to others: parents, relatives, those who care for the child. If they, however, reach the decision that the infant's life is not worth living then it may be taken. Professor Mitchell amply illustrates this philosophical view of the status of infants in his chapter. The BMA report notes and rejects this philosophical theory ' ... that would regard young infants as replaceable members of the series of potential persons' (page 45). It is based on a theoretical postulate: that no being without the present capacities to exercise the typical mental, rational abilities of a person is to be counted a person. Considerable effort has been devoted in contemporary moral philosophy to defending this postulate, but it may easily be seen why reflective medical practitioners should wish to reject it. It goes against a good deal of our normal thinking about what counts as homicide and against much legal thought and practice. Moreover, to any one engaged in the practicalities of decisions about when and when not to act to save and prolong life, it appears suspiciously theoretical.

Consider one of the most significant attempts to argue for this postulate of the un-personhood of infants: Michael Tooley's 'Abortion and Infanticide'.[10] This maintains that any duty not to kill infants must be grounded on *one* thing, namely the right to life that infants enjoy. However, Tooley also maintains that all rights must be based on corresponding desires, so that a being's rights cannot be violated unless some corresponding desire is frustrated. Since infants have no self-conscious awareness of themselves as continuing beings they have no desire to live. They cannot then have a right to life, so we have no duty not to kill them; only indirect considerations (such as causing pain and distress to the infant and others) might make the killing of an infant wrong. What is distinctive about this argument is the way it is embedded in an attempt to give a theoretically unified account of our moral judgments. Thus duties not to kill rest on only one thing: independently establishable rights on the part of potential victims. The possession of rights rests on one thing: desires. These affirmations will strike many unbiased readers as oversimplifications and they are unlikely to have any sympathy with them unless moved by the same theoretical concerns that influence Tooley. And here we must note a cultural fashion that has dictated the way that much, though not all, contemporary moral philosophy has been written. It is based on the premise that the task of moral philosophy must be to construct a theory for morality, one which will discover a relatively small number of principles from which all worthwhile moral judgments will follow. This entails searching for the lowest common denominator in terms of which rights and wrongs, benefits and harms can be expressed. It brings with it the attitude of the reformer: much ordinary moral thought is bound to need reshaping in the light of an adequate theory. Our ordinary moral judgments are so many 'intuitions' which need to be tested against theory. The 'intuitions' that do not fit in with the rest of our theory will be dismissed as unreliable. This is precisely what Tooley is proposing for our 'intuition' that we have a duty not to kill babies.

Now all the various elements of Tooley's approach to the morality of killing infants are open to philosophical questioning: the desire for moral theory,[11] the account of why killing is wrong,[8] the doctrine about the nature of rights.[12] Professor

Mitchell's chapter offers further criticism of the view that infants are not persons and indicates the range of philosophical opinion on just why and when human life becomes valuable. What will strike the medical practitioner as odd about Tooley's approach is that theory and abstract argument are being used to cloud an ordinary moral judgment that human infants are inherently worthy of respect and care. It is the bias towards theory that will no doubt appear sinister, and he may well judge that philosophical moralising of this sort is not aimed at elucidating and exploring our ordinary moral judgments but at playing a game of its own. While not all philosophers by any means share the theoretical drives that govern so much moral philosophy at present, it must be admitted that moral philosophy is a subject which has a particular institutional setting, its own fashions and biases. We must accept that these factors can mean that moral philosophy is very often not geared to searching out and producing practical wisdom.[13] In my own view, the particular institutional constraints, fashions, and so on, governing English-speaking moral philosophy of the 1980s have led to a good deal of practical unwisdom. If you want to find frequent examples of bad practical judgment, fantasy and nonsense, the moral philosophy shelves of a university library are among the best places to look.

No doubt it was the thought that the philosophical criticism of the killing/letting die distinction is driven by an impractical concern to propagate a theory (in particular a consequentialist moral theory). And that could explain why the BMA working party felt it so easy to reject this criticism. This was a mistake, for many of the important criticisms of killing/letting die are not moved by a hopeless concentration on the abstract demands of theory. They start from some firm judgments that ordinary moral agents make and which are enshrined in law. We know that killers can kill by inaction and neglect. We know that an intention to take life can be effected by refusing to provide the necessities of life to one who is too helpless to help himself. In considering the difference I allege to exist between the contemporary philosophical defence of killing babies and infants and the contemporary philosophical scepticism about the utility of a killing/letting die distinction, we see an important task for any critical medical ethics that is to be taken seriously by doctors: it has to find a way of distinguishing practical wisdom from unwisdom in the contribution of moral philosophy. In the case of a group of doctors considering the ethics of an area of their practice, the philosopher must be engaged from the start. He must be present to question and engage with medical testimony from the beginning and to see his own abstractions refined in the light of what makes sense to the moral agents involved in the practice. What some call 'philosophical' or 'critical medical ethics' is not a subbranch of philosophy, but an enterprise philosophers must pursue with the aid of doctors and others who are involved in the business of medicine.

In seeking to say something about the relation between moral philosophy and medical judgment, I have not discussed the substantive question of what might justify the homicidal acts which are performed in the care of handicapped infants. The principle that infants as such are not persons, and are not to enjoy the protection of our ethics and laws of homicide, is unlikely to commend itself. We know that the new born infant possesses potentially all the qualities that will make him worthy of the title 'human person' and of the respect for his life that goes with that. We know that he is one and the same being as the later adult he will grow into; that he and that adult are but two stages in the life of a single enduring substance. On these grounds we will judge that, if he will enjoy the protection of laws and principles forbidding homicide later in his life, he must enjoy them now. He cannot be viewed as a detached existent. He carries his future with him because we see him as a stage in the existence of a historical, enduring being (see Professor Mitchell's chapter and Kenny[14]). This might suggest that what lies behind our horror of baby killing is what Devine describes as a 'species principle' for fixing the scope of who is to be protected by our laws of homicide.[8] All those who are born as members of the human species are entitled to equal protection, regardless of other facts about them, such as their expected quality of life. Professor Mitchell hints at a species principle for homicide in his chapter. If the species principle is the right one and the duty not to kill it lays down applies with equal strictness to all cases, then the killings evident in paediatric practice surely count as unjustified homicide – that is, murder. In between Tooley's dismissal of the notion that killing infants is ever inherently wrong and the implications of an unqualified and rigorously interpreted species principle lies the use of the 'potentiality principle' to delimit the scope of homicide.[8] This tells us that all those who possess either actually or potentially the capacities of persons count as persons and are to enjoy the protection of restraints on homicide accordingly. The potentiality principle would appear to be at work in the judgments of paediatricians whose selective 'non-treatment' of malformed infants the BMA is prepared to endorse. They affirm, according to the BMA, the 'threshold conception of the quality of life' (page 46), defined previously as the hope that the infant will have a life that could reasonably be called the life of a person, involving at a minimum the capacity to appreciate human love and contact (pages 35–36).

How might we decide as a society whether a species principle, a potentiality principle, or some combination of both was the right one to use in marking out the distinction between justified and unjustified homicides in medical practice? This is not a question that we can hand over to either doctors or philosophers working in isolation. Any answer to the question will have to be based on argument and reflection, which must inevitably involve philosophical considerations. It will also have to draw on the experience of those who care for human beings whose quality of life is at the margins of personal existence. However, the necessary public debate on this issue cannot even begin unless it is acknowledged, both inside and outside the medical profession, that homicidal acts regularly occur within such areas as paediatric practice and that they therefore require some kind of social sanction and regulation. It is one more sad aspect of the killing/letting die distinction that its use prevents that acknowledgment.

When we turn from the BMA document to Professor Leenen's chapter and the Dutch debate he describes, we note with admiration the openness of Dutch medicine in setting out the fact that modern medical practice desires to kill some patients in some circumstances. The BMA working party may have shown that some of this medically required killing is not really necessary with the right kind of terminal care. But it singularly fails to disprove that none of it is required by apparently accepted strands of medical practice. The Dutch experience points also to what must follow from this admission (when it finally comes); society must then ask itself whether it wants to redefine its traditional conception of homicide and suicide to allow for medical killing in appropriate circumstances or, on the other hand, reinforce this conception at the cost of reining in modern developments in medical practice. Where statute and case law on homicide are not clear, then either option must involve setting our legislators the task of giving social policy on these matters a clear shape. Once again the Netherlands has shown us the way.

Is statute and case law on homicide, and particularly homicide in medical practice, clear? One thing that is evident about it is that it is not so wedded to the distinction between foresight and intention as the BMA. Accepted legal definitions of murder prescribe some 'malice aforethought' or appropriate *mens rea* before an act can count as murder. Yet case law has developed to the point where a jury will be allowed to infer that an agent intended his victim's death when, even though it is not desired, 'the result [death] is a virtually certain consequence of the act, and the actor knows that it is a virtually certain consequence'.[2] This fact about the definition of intent in law throws an ironic light on the BMA's reference to the law's 'deep seated adherence to intent rather than consequences alone' (page 68) in assessing the nature of actions. One thing an ethics of medical killing, or of homicide in general, needs to face is how far the homicidal consequences of decisions can be described as unintended when it is also admitted that these consequences can be foreseen with some certainty and are voluntarily accepted. Needless to say the BMA report does not explore this point, which happens to be the subject of intense controversy in philosophical discussions of the ethics of homicide (see Kuhse[7]). It indicates once more that English law is less enamoured of the killing/letting die distinction than doctors appear to be if the BMA correctly reflects the current wisdom of the profession.

When we turn to euthanasia and killing in medical practice we can find evidence to support the judgment that contemporary law is in need of greater consistency in its treatment of medical and non-medical assistance to acts of suicide. Recent cases involving infants selected for non-treatment also suggest that more needs to be done to give our law in this area some clear definition. They point indeed to a movement in our law towards the view, obviously implicit in parts of medical practice, that killing is not in all circumstances a harm to someone. Readers are referred to Kennedy for a detailed account of these matters.[15]

Society cannot, surely, leave the determination of the scope and limits of the range of justified homicide in clinical practice, or of justified assistance in suicide, to doctors acting in isolation. These are matters for social policy and the profession naturally has an important contribution to make. For the reasons outlined, the BMA report on euthanasia offers only a limited contribution from the profession to the making of adequate policy in this area.

## Notes and references

1 British Medical Association. Euthanasia: report of the working party to review the British Medical Association's guidance on euthanasia. London, BMA, 1988.

2 J C Smith and B Hogan. Criminal law (6th edition). London, Butterworths, 1988.

3 Peter Byrne. Review of the year 1 AIDS: the ethical, social and legal issues. In: Peter Byrne (ed). Health, rights and resources: King's College Studies 1987–8. London, King Edward's Hospital Fund for London, 1988, pages 11–34.

4 Roy Porter and Dorothy Porter. AIDS: law, liberty and public health. In: Peter Byrne (ed). Health, rights and resources: King's College Studies 1987–8. London, King Edward's Hospital Fund for London, 1988, pages 76–99.

5 Ruth Faden and others. A history and theory of informed consent. New York, Oxford University Press, 1986.

6 M Somerville. Consent to medical care. Ottawa, Law Reform Commission of Canada, 1980.

7 Helga Kuhse. The sanctity of life doctrine in medicine: a critique. Oxford, Clarendon Press, 1987.

8 P Devine. The ethics of homicide. Ithaca, New York, Cornell University Press, 1978.

9 Linacre Centre. Euthanasia and clinical practice: trends, principles and alternatives. The report of a working party (Chairman: Rev John Mahoney). London, Linacre Centre, 1982.

10 Michael Tooley. Abortion and infanticide. Philosophy and Public Affairs, 2, 1972, pages 137–165. The argument was subsequently enlarged upon in Tooley's book of the same title (Oxford, Clarendon Press, 1983).

11 Bernard Williams. Ethics and the limits of moral theory. London, Fontana, 1985.

12 Alan Richard White. Rights. Oxford, Clarendon Press, 1984.

13 Conversations with a colleague at King's College London, Dr Raimond Gaita, have brought this point home to me, though I have no doubt that he could express it better.

14 Anthony Kenny. Abortion and the taking of human life. In: Peter Byrne (ed). Medicine in contemporary society: King's College Studies 1986–7. London, King Edward's Hospital Fund for London, 1987, pages 84–98.

15 Ian Kennedy. R v Arthur, Re B, and the severely disabled new-born baby. In: Ian Kennedy (ed). Treat me right. Oxford, Clarendon Press, 1988, pages 154–175.

# The value of human life

Basil Mitchell

The philosopher-theologian, Baron von Hügel, in one of his delightful letters to his niece makes a distinction between the first and second clearness. He writes, 'Nothing in philosophy, still more in religion, should ever be attempted in and with the first clearness – what for example, journalists are content with, and have to be content with – but in and with the second clearness which only comes after that first cheery clarity has gone and has been succeeded by a dreary confusion and obtuseness of mind. Only this second clearness rising up, like something in no wise one's own, from the depth of one's subconsciousness, only this is any good in such great matters.'[1] Now I have to confess that on the important but difficult issues surrounding the value of human life, I find myself somewhere between von Hügel's two clearnesses and I fear that, as a result, much dreary confusion and obtuseness of mind will be apparent in my remarks.

That human life is valuable is among the most incontestable of moral platitudes. It is not surprising, therefore, that it figures among the 'universal values' that, according to Professor Herbert Hart, are acknowledged to some extent in all societies. One reason why this is so, is that no society could survive for long which regarded it as a matter of indifference whether its members lived or died. Recognition of a prohibition upon killing is a necessary condition of social existence. But, as Hart himself points out, 'it is perhaps misleading to say that social morality, so far as it secures these things [universal values of which safety of life is one], is of value because they are required for the preservation of society. On the contrary, the preservation of any particular society is of value because among other things it secures for human beings, some measure of these universal values.'[2] It is true no doubt that no society could survive which permitted its members to kill one another or neglect one another for personal advantage, but long-lived and stable societies have tolerated and even encouraged such practices as duelling, the vendetta, infanticide, sacrificial killing; and many societies have regarded as of comparatively little value the lives of aliens and of racial minorities.

Hart is plainly right, then, in holding that the universality of this value is not to be established by its social necessity. For a society would not be worth living in, if it did not attach a high value to human life. But that leaves unanswered the question: what makes it a universal value if it is one and, indeed, to what extent or in what sense is it a universal value?

Certain obvious answers suggest themselves:

1. We want to live, at least most of us most of the time want to live. Any moral system which derives its principles from the universalising of our preferences will therefore number among its principles a prohibition on taking life. Willing, as we do, that we ourselves should not be killed, we are bound also to will that other people should not be killed either.

2. Life is a necessary condition of all other good things. It is in this sense a fundamental value and this is one reason, perhaps, and indeed may be the chief reason, why it is so widely valued.

3. The value we are concerned with is that of *human* life and the prohibition upon taking human life reflects, arguably, an estimate of human life as worthy of a unique respect. Views may differ as to what it is in human beings that commands such unique respect, but characteristics such as rationality, self-determination, consciousness, have been emphasised, especially in the philosophical tradition deriving from Kant and the Enlightenment.

4. That particular tradition is somewhat severely rationalist but it is not incompatible with another strain in Western thought of a more romantic kind. This would stress the mysteriousness and inexhaustibility of human beings. Respect is due not only to what we can clearly comprehend and assess in people, but also to what eludes and, indeed, transcends our understanding of them. The point is well put by Professor Mahoney. 'There is an element of sheer mystery about human existence which lays

a claim upon men to reverence and respect it, to foster it and not to destroy it. Even on the most ordinary grounds, apart from any religious considerations, human life is a deep mystery ... at the heart of each one of us in an intractable, perhaps impenetrable, personal core.'[3]

All these considerations are likely to appeal to those who have been reared in what may be broadly called the Western ethical tradition. Nevertheless, this appearance of a consensus is to some extent misleading as becomes evident when attention is directed to the scope and practical implications of recognising this value.

It is possible to interpret three at least of the considerations I have just mentioned in a somewhat minimalist fashion as giving only a qualified or restricted value to much of human life:

1. Thus we all want to live – most of us most of the time. But some of us some of the time do not want to live, or can envisage circumstances in which we would not want to live. So we want to live, it may be said, only conditionally, and it would seem that any universal prohibition of killing based upon our preferences would have to be less than absolute. It is at least arguable that by this criterion suicide, euthanasia, and infanticide, would not be ruled out if, in a particular case, the outcome of asking the question 'in such and such circumstances would I wish to live?' were to be in the negative. (Of course, this would not necessarily be the end of the matter from this broadly utilitarian standpoint. Professor R M Hare, for example, would insist that the further question be raised whether we need in practice a comparatively strict rule governing these things.)

2. It is possible, indeed tempting, to argue that if respect for human life is properly based on such characteristic features of human life as rationality, self-determination, capacity for social relationships and so on, it extends only to those human lives which actually manifest these characteristics. Account may, no doubt, be taken of the potentiality to develop these things or of someone's having once possessed them, but a special case has to be made out for any such extension.

3. Similarly it may seem reasonable to argue that, if life is to be valued as the necessary condition of the enjoyment of everything else that is valuable, its value is essentially instrumental. It is to be valued because of the experience and activities it makes possible, and that means *to the extent that* it makes them possible. No doubt there will always be a strong presumption that life is valuable, but that presumption is capable of being rebutted if the quality of life declines sufficiently.

The possibility of these divergent interpretations of what had at first sight seemed a platitude points to underlying differences of a philosophical kind. And recent debate about the issue has indeed revealed sharply differing conceptions of the nature of man, and has directed attention quite explicitly to their contrasting ethical implications. An extreme example is provided by B F Skinner's book, *Beyond Freedom and Dignity*. Skinner deliberately rejects the conception of man as an autonomous, self-determining individual which makes him particularly worthy of respect. He responds to C S Lewis's despairing cry, 'Man is being abolished', by asserting bluntly that his abolition has long been overdue. 'Autonomous man', he goes on, 'is a device used to explain what we cannot explain in any other way. He has been constructed from our ignorance and, as our understanding increases, the very stuff of which he is composed vanishes. Science does not dehumanise man, it dehomunculises him. To man as man, we readily say "good riddance". Only by dispossessing him, can we turn to the real cause of human behaviour. Only then can we turn from the inferred to the observed, from the miraculous to the natural, from the inaccessible to the manipulable. Rationality and self-determination are thus dissolved into complex patterns of reinforcement, and the mysteriousness of human personality becomes nothing but a function of our ignorance.'[4]

Skinner's thesis depends on a somewhat crude form of neo-behaviourist psychology which is not now widely accepted by academic psychologists. Its chief interest in the present context is that it illustrates in a particularly striking way the relationship between the value placed on human life and the view that is held about the human person. Skinner's title is here revealing: *Beyond Freedom and Dignity*. Human dignity is eroded along with human freedom.

A somewhat less extreme critique of traditional claims for
the unique value of human life is presented by Helga Kuhse
and Peter Singer in their book, *Should the Baby Live? The
Problem of Handicapped Infants.* They direct a head-on
assault against the Western consensus of which I spoke earlier.
They write:

> We shall show that the doctrine of the sanctity of human life,
> as understood in the Western tradition since Christianity
> prevailed, is not in any sense a fundamental tenet of a
> civilised society. There have been innumerable societies
> which have not shared the Western belief in the sanctity of
> human life, though many of these societies had as strong a
> claim to the label 'civilised' as our own.[5]

They take as their chief illustration infanticide which was
widely accepted, for example, in the Graeco-Roman world of
antiquity and in 18th century Japan. These and other examples,
they claim, are enough to show that infanticide is compatible
with a stable, well-organised human society;[6] and the evidence
they adduce does show, I think, that the principle of the
sanctity of human life is not a universal value in the sense of one
whose general acceptance is a necessary condition of the
survival of a society or indeed of a civilised society, if that
expression is broadly enough understood.

This point was brought home to me personally when I had in
my graduate class a Chinese girl from Hong Kong who was a
Christian convert. Whenever, as quite often happened, someone from Europe or North America mentioned respect for
human life as a universal value characteristic of all human
societies, she would intervene and say: 'Not so. In the classical
Chinese tradition in which I was brought up, we were taught
respect for parents, respect for teachers, respect for ancestors
and for duly constituted authority, but the conception of
respect due to the individual human being as such does not
exist in that culture.' She insisted that we Westerners all take it
so much for granted because of the unacknowledged influence
of Christian belief upon our system of values; and this is also
the explanation that Kuhse and Singer give for the prevalence
of this conviction in the Western world. They write: 'The
traditional principle of the sanctity of human life is the
outcome of some seventeen centuries of Christian domination

of Western thought and cannot be rationally defended.'[7] It seems obvious to them that it cannot be rationally defended, not only because they reject the religious beliefs upon which they believe it to rest, but because it attaches moral significance to something which, plainly, can have no intrinsic importance – the bare fact that an individual belongs to the human race. This, they say, is the error of 'speciesism'. Species membership might be morally relevant, they argue, if it were a reliable indicator of capacities that are directly relevant to moral worth; but whatever you list as the characteristics of humanity in virtue of which human beings are worthy of a unique respect, there are members of the human species that do not possess them. The anencephalic child, to take the most obvious example, never attains consciousness and can never respond to other human beings; it lacks rationality or power of self-determination.

The more rational procedure, Kuhse and Singer claim, is to base one's moral principles, not upon arbitrary and irrelevant factors like membership of a particular biological species, but upon the actual possession of respect-worthy characteristics. They suggest, as a basic minimum, self-awareness and a sense of the future. It follows, of course, and they accept, that normal babies do not qualify in the first few months of life, unless we are prepared to ascribe a significance to their *potentiality* for rational existence. The whole tenor of their discussion so far has been to suggest that mere potentiality is not enough, but they are prepared to ascribe some value, although not an overriding value, to the creation of additional human life, and this is enough to provide at least a *prima facie* case for not killing young babies. This case is capable of being strengthened in particular instances by other considerations. The baby may because of its circumstances have potential for a particularly happy and worthwhile existence; it may be very much wanted by its parents or by others and so on.

It would be possible to reinforce this line of argument by familiar utilitarian considerations. There is, from this general standpoint, no objection in principle to infanticide; nevertheless, widespread condonation of infanticide might encourage the killing of babies from motives of temporary convenience or passing irritation. To avoid this it might be wise to adopt a general prohibition of the practice so long as genuine and justifiable exceptions (of which, on Kuhse's and Singer's assumption, there would be many) were readily accepted. It might be thought that similar utilitarian considerations could be developed on the other side in terms of the risk that a greater acceptance of infanticide would weaken the protection afforded in our society to the lives of adults, especially to those who are temporarily or permanently disabled. But this is a pattern of reasoning that Kuhse and Singer explicitly reject. They write:

> It is sometimes said that if we start to kill severely handicapped infants, we will end up threatening severely disabled adults as well. To allow infanticide before the onset of self-awareness, however, cannot threaten anyone who is in a position to worry about it. Anyone able to understand what it is to live or die must already be a person and has the same right to life as all the rest of us.[8]

But what of those who eventually lose all their ability to be self-aware, and their sense of the future? Will they not lose also their right to life since they no longer possess the characteristics upon which that right depends? No, 'because once a being with a sense of the future exists, that being can have an interest in her or his future existence. This interest should be respected.'

Now the importance of Kuhse's and Singer's position is that it radically challenges the Western ethical tradition, and it does so by probing the consensus that appears to exist, and suggesting that those who subscribe to it rely in fact on divergent philosophical theories not all of which, when carefully examined, actually support the principle. More specifically what they claim to show is that in our society Christians and Humanists wrongly suppose themselves to agree in acknowledging a principle of the sanctity of life, and to disagree only about the considerations that justify the principle. Whereas in fact, they urge, as soon as the arguments upon which the principle appears to rest are made explicit, it becomes apparent that the principle as traditionally received can be supported only by explicitly theological argument; and that the non-theological arguments which have been thought also to support it would in fact only support something very much weaker, which is compatible with, for example, the fairly widespread practice of infanticide.

When this Humanist alternative is spelt out in detail by

Kuhse and Singer it is likely to be profoundly shocking not only to Christians but to Humanists also. The practical implications are such that our moral intuitions are strongly inclined to repudiate them. Kuhse and Singer, for their part, will admit that this is so, and explain this fact by calling attention to the enormous extent to which our moral intuitions have for centuries been formed by Christianity. This being the case, they will argue, we cannot simply trust our intuitions to adjudicate between the theoretical alternatives presented to us. Those intuitions themselves are hopelessly compromised.

But they do, of course, appeal to intuition themselves. Part of their strategy consists in drawing out the implications, as they see them, of the traditional Christian view and inviting us to reject them. It means, for example, that we have an absolute duty, to preserve the life of anencephalic children and yet it is obvious, is it not, that we can have no such duty? We do not, surely, on reflection find that we attach a value, let alone a supreme value, to mere biological life that has no potentiality for the development of what is characteristically human.

I mentioned at an earlier stage the temptation to confine the value of human life to those lives or those periods of a particular life in which the characteristically human qualities are plainly manifested. This is precisely what Kuhse and Singer do. Infanticide is in principle allowable, in their view, because babies are not yet persons, and the elderly demented, who are no longer persons, have a right to life because, and presumably only because, they wanted it when they were still persons. This way of looking at people has the effect of making them, as it were, channels through which activities and experiences flow, the latter being the only things which are properly valued in themselves. But this is open to a serious objection. Whenever we are deeply attached to people (and love is one of the chief activities and experiences we value), we cannot think of them in this way. The person is, indeed, most fully *manifested* in the exercise and enjoyment of his or her capacities but what we love is a human being whose identity is continuous from birth to death. We do not, when we love, take a section through a person's life – here is something that is conscious and rational and responsive to others, and to be loved on account of these attributes for so long as they are apparent – but rather commit ourself to the person as someone who endures throughout all life's vicissitudes. This is memorably expressed in the Prayer Book marriage service: 'for better or for worse, in sickness and in health, to love and to cherish until death do us part'. Someone's identity as the person we love does not fluctuate with the degree of intensity or effectiveness with which he or she displays characteristically human attributes. Similarly, small babies are full members of the human race, that 'natural kind' whose fully developed members are characteristically conscious, rational and capable of responding in love to one another; and we do not, and surely should not, withhold from babies the respect we show to human beings until we can be sure that they will in fact become fully rational individuals, self-determining, and so forth. Indeed, it is essential to the development of babies that they are from the beginning treated as fully human and encouraged to trust their parents and others who have to deal with them. They become persons by being treated as persons.

The charge of speciesism, which Kuhse and Singer level against the Western ethical tradition rests on their claim that it is merely arbitrary to regard a severely retarded human being as deserving of greater respect than a healthy animal on the grounds that it is biologically human. They contend that pigs, cows and chickens have a greater capacity to relate to others, better ability to communicate, and far more curiosity than the most severely retarded humans. But it is not arbitrary to take account of what human beings as such have it in them to be. '*Homo sum: humani nihil a me alienum puto*' ('I am a man, and I count nothing alien to me') as the poet Terence wrote.

Yet there is a genuine dilemma when brought face to face with hard cases. The sort of cases which present the problems are familiar enough – the ones where our reflective judgment or intuition would be that there are good reasons for not prolonging a life. In looking for a rationale for such intuitions we are liable to be forced in one or other of two directions, neither of which is immediately satisfying. One direction is the assessment of the quality of life. The question to ask is: Is the likely quality of life of this individual baby or old person such as to justify trying to keep him or her alive? Kuhse and Singer would be entirely happy with this question, but that of course is the rub, because they are also happy with direct euthanasia in such cases and they are prepared to envisage further extensions which many of us would not tolerate. What then, we wonder, are we letting ourselves in for if we ask this particular question? The other direction leads us away from any such question about the quality of life. Indeed we are forbidden to ask it. The matter is discussed with exemplary clarity in the Linacre Centre's report *Euthanasia and Clinical Practice*. The report insists on 'the fundamentally important distinction between, on the one hand, withholding treatment because one does not consider a patient as having a worthwhile life (and we reject the view that such global assessments of quality of life are either possible or appropriate), and on the other hand withholding treatment because the treatment is of too little benefit relative to the risks or burdens involved.'[9] The report emphasises the importance of recognising when a patient is dying, at which point the entire concern of the medical team switches from the attempt to prolong life to the need to enable the patient to die well. There is here the sense of cooperating with a natural process, an element that is missing entirely in Kuhse's and Singer's approach, and I welcome that emphasis. But what of those who are not dying but who suffer from a severely incapacitating condition? The Linacre Centre's report is committed to the principle that only strictly medical judgments should be made in such a case. That is to say, the only question under consideration should be the burden and benefits of a specific treatment. Will the benefits, in medical terms, of a proposed treatment be worthwhile in relation to the burdens which that same treatment imposes? In such a formulation no reference is made to the patient's overall quality of life in so far as it is not affected or modified by the proposed treatment. In other words, it is proper, from this point of view, to conclude that the likely improvement in the patient's condition from the treatment is not enough to warrant the burdens imposed by the treatment, but not to conclude that the patient's condition is such that it is not worthwhile trying to improve it. In the first case, the pros and cons of a particular treatment are considered; in the second case, a global assessment of the quality of life of the individual is made and this the authors wish to rule out as illegitimate.

It can be seen why the authors of the report formulate the question in such a way as to avoid estimating the overall quality of life of the patient. They suspect that, as soon as we even raise the question 'is the patient's quality of life such that it would be better for the patient not to be alive?' we are committed in principle to the policy that Kuhse and Singer advocate. 'We ought instead, then', they insist, 'to acknowledge an absolute prohibition on the taking of innocent human lives; and "human", quite simply means belonging to the human race.' On this they are entirely clear and explicit. They write:

> for a person is a substantial human being with his own identity which he has as an individual of a particular species. In our case the species is human being. Having named an individual human being we use the name with the same reference so long as it is the same human being we are talking about. A human being is a person because the kind to which he belongs is characterised by rational nature ... One is a person just by being of this kind and that does indeed import a tremendous dignity.[10]

There is not, then, any possibility of dealing with the anencephalic or the irreversibly unconscious by claiming that they are not in any relevant sense human. The decision to give them only palliative treatment in such cases, must be based on some other consideration. For reasons already mentioned, the consideration that the patient's condition is such that there is for him or her no interest in continued life, is ruled out as illegitimate. Hence the recourse to the language of benefits or burdens of the treatment, or alternatively to the claim that treatment would in such cases be 'futile'.

And yet, perhaps, this interpretation of the report is too hasty, for it says:

> We do not deny that judgements which can (but need not) be called quality of life judgements do enter into the process of medical decision-making ... The doctor makes some sort of comparison – weighing is too simple a metaphor – between the benefits and the risks and burdens for the patient that will or may accrue from the specific treatment under consideration. *And this comparison is inevitably made against the background of the patient's present and likely condition and prognosis* [my italics]. So the question being asked, implicitly, can be put thus: given his present 'quality of life' are the burdens of this (expensive or time-consuming

or painful or disfiguring or undignified ... ) medical
treatment worth enduring, in view of (a) the probable
'quality of his life' while undergoing it and (b) the probable
quality of his life if and when the treatment is completed?[11]

It is not clear that this question, which is indeed the right
question to ask, conforms to the requirement they have
previously laid down that only the benefits and burdens *of the
treatment* should be considered. Suppose, for example, that the
burdens of the treatment were negligible and the benefits were
more than sufficient to offset them, the likely quality of life
upon completion of the treatment might yet be such that it
would not be worth while embarking upon it. Would not one,
in such a case, be judging that the patient's quality of life, quite
apart from the nature and effects of the proposed intervention,
made any but palliative treatment futile?

If this is so, the question remains whether those who make
such a judgment are, whether they like it or not, committed to
approval in principle of euthanasia and, therefore, infanticide.
Have they, by allowing 'quality of life' to enter at all into their
deliberations, embarked upon the slippery slope down which
Kuhse and Singer's argument invites them? The answer is
clearly 'no'. Kuhse and Singer's argument for infanticide only
works within the crudely utilitarian framework they have
adopted, with its characteristic neglect of the essential continuity
of personal life and its fundamental mysteriousness. The
Western ethical tradition starts from a very different position,
in which these considerations are given full weight. The fact
that, in certain extreme cases, the individual's quality of life
may be judged so poor as to make it pointless to keep him or
her alive does not in the least imply that quality of life is
normally the sole criterion to apply in deciding questions of
life and death. It shows only that acceptance of the principle of
the sanctity of human life in its traditional form does not
relieve us of the burden of decisions in difficult cases, where
what is at stake is the proper interpretation of the principle
itself or how to relate it to other principles, such as those of
beneficence and non-maleficence.

There is a complexity about such cases which makes reliance
upon personal judgment in the end unavoidable. And it would
only be after detailed examination of many such cases that
one could begin to approach von Hügel's 'second clearness'.

Notes and references

1 G Greene (ed). Letters from Baron Friedrich von Hügel to a niece. J M Dent, 1928, page 74.

2 H L A Hart. Law, liberty and morality. Oxford, Oxford University Press, 1963, page 70.

3 John Mahoney. Bioethics and belief: religion and medicine in dialogue. London, Sheed and Ward, 1984, page 41.

4 B F Skinner. Beyond freedom and dignity. Harmondsworth, Penguin, 1973, page 191.

5 Helga Kuhse and Peter Singer. Should the baby live? The problem of handicapped infants. Oxford, Oxford University Press, 1985, page 98.

6 See 5 above, page 108.

7 See 5 above, page 122.

8 See 5 above, page 138.

9 Linacre Centre. Euthanasia and clinical practice: trends, principles and alternatives. The report of a working party (Chairman: Rev. John Mahoney). London, Linacre Centre, 1982, page 60.

10 See 9 above, page 28.

11 See 9 above, page 30.

# Abortion, embryo research and fetal transplantation: their moral interrelationships

Sophie Botros

Recent controversies surrounding abortion and the use of fetal material both for non-therapeutic research[1] and for transplantation (fetal brain cells, for instance, have been transplanted into the brain of patients with Parkinson's disease),[2] make it timely that we explore the moral interrelationships between these procedures.

Three distinct positions may be adopted towards them. Each may be regarded either as morally permissible in all circumstances, as morally impermissible in all circumstances, or as morally permissible only in some circumstances.

Abortion, for instance, may be considered impermissible except where the mother's life is at risk or where the pregnancy is a consequence of rape. Current British abortion legislation however permits abortion until late in pregnancy[3] on more liberal grounds:

1. Where a continued pregnancy involves risk of injury to the mother's physical or mental health (without necessarily endangering her life) or to that of any existing children of her family, greater than if the pregnancy were terminated.
2. Where there is a substantial risk that if the child were born it would suffer severe congenital disability.[4]

With embryo research, a morally relevant factor is often thought to be the source from which the embryos are obtained. Thus some writers consider research using embryos whose creation has been specially facilitated for that purpose morally impermissible, however enticing the ultimate benefits. They may however support research using embryos left over after *in vitro* fertilisation (the process by which human ova are fertilised *in vitro*, the resultant embryos grown for a period in the laboratory, and then one or more implanted into a woman). An analogous distinction is made by the British Medical Association in its guidelines concerning fetal transplantation, which is considered morally permissible if the prior abortion is performed for reasons unconnected with the subsequent transplantation. But, though her motive might be impeccably altruistic, a woman is absolutely forbidden from seeking an abortion in order that fetal material might be used to cure a sufferer from, for example, Parkinsonism.[5]

A more uncompromising position is adopted, however, by those who warn that embryo research and fetal transplantation are, unlike abortion, situated upon a 'slippery slope' at the bottom of which lie atrocities such as the Nazis perpetrated. Wishing therefore to ban these medical procedures altogether, they make the following claim (stated here only with respect to embryo research since this will be the focus of my interest):

(T) Embryo research is always immoral, and hence never morally permissible, whereas abortion is sometimes morally permissible.

The typical attack upon this position,[6] the validity of which will be my main concern, has two variants. It may be argued that we cannot consistently object to embryo research, whether upon the spare embryos of *in vitro* fertilisation (IVF) or upon those specially created for that purpose, if we hold that abortion is ever morally permissible or, less strongly, if we accept current liberal abortion laws. Moreover, it will be added, if we accept current legislation which allows abortion late into pregnancy, we can hardly object, as does Professor Ian Kennedy in a celebrated article[7], to research upon embryos after, let alone before, 14 days.

This attack is of the general form: you hold that embryo research is x, and that x is morally impermissible, but abortion is also x (or, at least, if embryo research is x, then abortion also is), hence you cannot consistently both object to embryo research and support abortion. If successful, this attack would only rule out holding both positions simultaneously; it would not show which of them, if either, is correct. Nevertheless, it would be enough, assuming x was the ground of the objection to embryo research, to undermine (T). For it entails that some part of (T) is false. On the other hand, as we shall see, to demonstrate that this thesis can consistently be maintained is not to uphold it.

What then is the characteristic of embryo research which, it is claimed, makes embryo research, unlike abortion, always morally impermissible? Professor Kennedy, a noted proponent[8] of (T), argues that research should never be allowed on embryos after they have achieved even limited 'humanness' because this transgresses 'a fundamental principle – that we may not use humans as means to an end but must respect them as ends in themselves'. Later, in outlawing research upon embryos even before they have reached this stage, he links their being 'used' with their being denied, in the interests of research, the possibility of further development,[9] and with their subsequent destruction. He clearly does not regard abortion as involving the use of the fetus and hence as warranting a similarly sweeping condemnation.

Now Kennedy, in alleging that researchers 'use' the embryo, has surely put his finger upon a quite fundamental aspect of our moral disquiet. But is this disquiet justified? Indisputably, researchers in some sense use the embryo. But do they really use it in a manner which is morally impermissible and, even if they do, may it not be claimed that abortion is equally open to this charge? To answer these questions we must clarify the meaning of the word 'use'.

Is the embryo 'used', for instance, because it is made use of? And if so, does the researcher make use of the embryo merely because he uses it as a tool to contribute to the advancement of his ends, or because his making use of it in this way leads to its death? Or, alternatively, is the embryo 'used' simply because it is killed to benefit others? If so, then of course the aborted[10] fetus is 'used' too since, though it is not killed to be made use of, the welfare of the mother or her other children is deemed to require its elimination.

The language of use is clearly Kantian. Indeed Kant regarded the moral prohibition upon 'using persons merely as means' as so fundamental that he enshrined it in his second formulation of the Categorical Imperative.[11] It is appropriate then to turn to Kant for a clarification of the above questions.

In the remaining sections, I will first show that it is a mistaken interpretation of Kant's formulation which, filtering down through popular consciousness, is responsible for the prevalent feeling that researchers, just because they make use of the embryo, are using it 'merely as a means', and thereby violating the Kantian imperative, whereas abortionists, because they do not make use of the fetus, escape that stricture. Hence the thesis (T) cannot be maintained on this ground.

I will then ask just what Kant does mean by his moral injunction not to use people 'merely as a means'. I try to show that, stripped to its essentials, it is a prohibition on overriding people's rights and interests without justification and that, thus clarified, it provides a sound basis, despite certain limitations, for the moral evaluation of conduct even towards people incapable of rational thought.

Before turning, however, to the question of whether (T)[12] might receive corroboration from this revised reading of Kant's prohibition, I demonstrate that just as (T) cannot be upheld by, so it is also immune to attack from, arguments which rest upon a flawed understanding of that prohibition. Typical of the latter is the following attempt to undermine (T)'s consistency: if embryos and fetuses are persons, then abortion, since it, like embryo research, eliminates fetuses for the benefit of others, involves using embryos and fetuses 'merely as a means' and hence is equally immoral. The failure of this argument, as I show, leaves even (T)'s consistency intact.

Given then the revised reading of Kant's prohibition, I next consider the requirements for upholding (T) as opposed just to defending its consistency. It is not sufficient that justifications are available to support abortion which cannot be adduced in favour of embryo research. These justifications must be powerful enough, if embryos and fetuses are considered to be persons, to absolve those who perform abortions from using the fetus 'merely as a means'. Moreover, there must be no independent, but equally defensible, justifications for embryo research for, if there were, embryo research would sometimes be morally permissible, which (T) denies. My remarks in this, and preceding sections, though directed toward embryo research, may be adapted to apply to fetal transplantation.

I next examine and dismiss a second moral position which might underlie the greater moral repugnance that is frequently felt about embryo research and fetal transplantation than about abortion:

> Abortion is immoral, and hence never permissible, but embryo research and fetal transplantation are still more immoral.

Finally I look at a problem which relates only to fetal transplantation. If abortion is held to be morally wrong, yet transplantation of fetal brain cells into the brains of sufferers with Parkinsonism really could cure their disease, what is the proper attitude to an immoral action that has a potential for good and, in particular, is it wrong to attempt to realise that good once the immoral action has unavoidably occurred? Although I will not offer much concrete guidance here, I hope to clarify the issues upon which the moral decisions turn.

It may seem that the following discussion of Kant's views will only be relevant to embryos and fetuses in so far as they are considered to be persons. This, of course, is a highly debatable question which I will not go into.[13] But even if they are not persons, Kant's approach may well supply a useful set of ideas with which to evaluate the ways in which we treat them and other non-persons, such as animals. This however is the topic for another occasion.

## 1. An attempt to uphold (T) and an attack on its consistency

### Kant: means and obstacles

Kant's discussion of the proper treatment of persons is found in chapter 2 of his *Groundwork of the Metaphysic of Morals* in the section entitled 'The Formula of the End in Itself'.[14] There, persons, in contrast with 'things' (animals and other 'non-rational' creatures), are said to possess an 'absolute' value or a value which is not conditional upon their utility. This value 'marks persons out as ends in themselves' or beings 'which ought not to be used merely as a means'.[15]

For Kant, then, it is because persons (unlike 'things') possess a value which transcends their utility that we must not value them only in so far as they are useful. Not to observe this prohibition is to 'use them merely as a means'.

The notion of valuing a person only in so far as she is of use is then central to the understanding of Kant's expression 'using a person merely as a means'. Indeed, reflection upon it, helps us to see (as few writers on Kant have seen)[16] that the Kantian notion of 'using a person merely as a means' is relatively independent of the more common notions of 'using someone as a means' or 'making use' of her.

For implicit in the idea of valuing a person only in so far as she is of use is the idea of not valuing her at all when she is not of use. Suppose then I value someone only in so far as she is of use. It follows that there are two kinds of situation in which to appraise my behaviour towards her. There is the question of how I treat her when she is of use and the question of how I treat her when she is not of use. But even when she is not of use, and so can no longer be used as a means or made use of, my conduct towards her still expresses a wrongful valuation of her – one that is conditional upon her utility – and thus counts, by Kantian standards, as 'using her merely as a means'.

That it is therefore impossible to escape Kant's strictures against using someone 'merely as a means' by pleading that we are not even using her as a means has, of course, immediate implications, as we shall see, for the moral comparison of embryo research and abortion. For these procedures differ precisely in that the one, but not the other, involves using the embryo or fetus as a means or making use of it.

Approaching, then, the notion of 'using a person merely as a means' through the less misleading idea of valuing her only in so far as she is of use, I shall now outline the different kinds of conduct that this merely conditional valuation of people typically leads to in the two main circumstances to which I have drawn attention.

If a person is of use to me, then my failure to recognise that her value transcends her utility will show itself in my making use of her either against her will or by deception (Kant's example is a false promise)[17] or, we might suppose, in a way that is grossly contrary to her interests, where she is incapable of realising it. (This last case, however, will require further discussion.) If embryo research involves using the embryo 'merely as a means' it will fall into this general category since, being of use, the embryo is, as Kant would put it, of 'relative value as a means'.[15]

If however a person is no longer of use to me then, if I value her only in so far as she is of use, I will typically abandon her. For, having neither inclination towards her nor need of her,[18] she does not even possess for me 'relative value as a means'. If she is an actual obstacle to my goals, my actions will purely depend upon how she impedes my interests. If, for instance, she is a colleague at work, and is spoiling my chances of promotion, then I may try to get her fired. If, however, her very existence stands in my way to some important goal, then I may even contemplate destroying her. In such 'attempts on the freedom of others', Kant asserts, we become 'violators of the rights of man'.[17] Moreover, he goes so far as to apply his strictures to suicide: 'But man is not a thing – not something to be used merely as a means ... hence I cannot dispose of man in my own person by maiming, spoiling or killing'. Clearly if abortion ever involves using the fetus 'merely as a means' it will fall into this second category since the aborted fetus, being of no use, even impeding other people's interests, is not even of 'relative value as a means'. The object is simply to dispose of it.

For Kant then, in using someone 'merely as a means', we may do so either because she is a *means* or because she is an *obstacle* to our goals. But only where she is a means to our goals do we actually *make use* of her. Hence to make use of someone, even where that also counts as using her 'merely as a means', is not, according to Kant, the only way we may use her 'merely as a means'. Of course, casting someone aside because she stands in our way is a means to an end. But since such a person does not herself serve us as a means, we use her 'merely as a means' without making use of her.

This point, as we have noted, is obscured by Kant's own wording of his second formulation, with its reference to 'means'. Yet, taken together with his view that we may make use of someone without using her 'merely as a means',[17] it blocks any appeal to Kant as support for morally condemning embryo researchers on grounds that they, unlike abortionists,[19] make use of the embryo. For making use of the embryo is neither necessary nor sufficient for using it 'merely as a means'.

*Kant: using a person merely as a means*

Though Kant, surprisingly, does not offer any necessary conditions for using a person 'merely as a means', he suggests, at different points in his text, two conditions which appear to be disjunctively sufficient. Both of these conditions refer directly to behaviour rather than to any attitude which might underlie it.

He first introduces such a condition in his discussion of false promises. I use a person 'merely as a means' and hence impermissibly, he writes, not because I 'make use' of her, but because I do so *when* she does not 'share the end of my action'. But if I have deliberately concealed from someone what I intend to do to her, she 'cannot possibly have agreed' to my action.[17] She cannot therefore 'share in the end of (my) action' and is hence used 'merely as a means'. Such is the position of someone to whom I have made a false promise.

But I could not have made a false promise to someone incapable of understanding or consenting to my intentions. Hence it might seem that using a person 'merely as a means' is a wrong I can only commit against one capable of consent. In failing to consult her, and thus to secure her agreement to my proposed treatment of her, I strike at her very essence as an autonomous being. I may also, especially if she is unaware of my intentions, and so cannot defend herself, harm her. But harming her is not intrinsic to using her 'merely as a means'. For, had she consented to my harming her for, say, other people's benefit, she would nevertheless have 'shared in the end of my action'.[20]

On this reading, then, it would be incoherent to condemn me for using someone 'merely as a means' if I could not even in principle have secured her agreement. (Suppose that, being very young or brain-damaged or in a coma, she is incapable of having views about and thus of making choices as to how I should treat her.)

Any claim, based upon the Kantian prohibition against using people 'merely as means', that embryo research is morally impermissible would thus immediately be undermined. It would not even be necessary to attack the status of embryos as persons, supposing it could be secured independently of their capacity to have opinions as to how they should be treated. Along with certain even more developed humans they would, whether persons or not, simply no longer qualify as candidates for being used 'merely as a means'.

But it would, I believe, be misleading to interpret Kant in this way. For he suggests elsewhere a much less narrowly focused account of what it is to use a person 'merely as a means'. On page 90, for instance, he writes that persons do not exist 'for arbitrary use by this or that will'. And again, on page 91, he states that being 'objects of reverence' they 'impose ... a limit on all arbitrary treatment of them'. On page 93 he asserts that persons, existing as 'ends in themselves', and not merely 'happening to be made ends' by us, 'constitute the supreme limiting condition of all subjective ends'.

Kant's point, I take it, is that a person's rights and interests set limits upon what I may properly do to her in the pursuit of my goals. It is by failing to acknowledge these constraints (and not, for instance, by any actual damage I may incidentally do her) that I use her 'merely as a means'. On this account, a person could not 'share in the end of (an) action' by which I violate her rights or run roughshod over her interests, since I thereby fail to treat her 'as an object of reverence'.

Of course, the interests of a person in full possession of her rational faculties will not simply be a narrow matter of her own welfare but will comprise all the purposes she might entertain. But we do not always have to consult a person to discover, and hence to respect, her rights and interests, even when the latter are thus widely construed. Moreover, only the most radical of contemporary writers would jib at the ascription to someone of rights and interests (in the narrower sense in which they are co-extensive with her welfare) just because she was incapable of any opinion as to how she was to be treated or what she wished to achieve.

Suppose, for instance, that a couple adopt a baby. At first they care for her, play with her, draw her into the family circle. Soon, however, the novelty of a new face wears off, and they begin to resent the financial and other sacrifices that keeping her demand. Without a thought for the emotional damage that this traumatic uprooting will wreak upon her, they callously return her to the adoption agency. Now the baby can hardly be described as having desires in the matter of whether or not she is to be sent back to the agency. Yet we could surely condemn the couple for failing to acknowledge that the baby's rights and interests impose limits upon what they may properly do to her, and thus for using her 'merely as a means'.

The most that can be extracted from Kant's discussion of false promises is this: to avoid using someone 'merely as a means', either when she is in full possession of her rational powers or when these are temporarily eclipsed, we must get (or wait until we can get) her agreement to our proposed treatment of her. But even this requires qualification. For, according to Kant, we do not necessarily use a person 'merely as a means' even if we act towards her in a way that is deliberately contrary to her wishes. For Kant, a person's desires or intentions may contravene the moral law even where they can be fulfilled without harming others. Wanting to commit suicide is, as we have seen, a case in point. But if it is in obedience to the moral law that we refuse to help someone commit suicide, or even deliberately resuscitate her against her wishes, we can hardly be described as subjecting her to our 'arbitrary will'. Therefore, we can hardly be accused of using her 'merely as a means'. But if acting contrary to a person's wishes is neither necessary nor sufficient for using her 'merely as a means' it hardly seems that we must exclude embryos as candidates for such treatment on grounds that they are incapable of having wishes that we might neglect or contravene.

## Limitations of Kant's account

Kant's notion of using someone 'merely as a means', even when explicated in terms of the failure to acknowledge the limits imposed upon our conduct by other people's rights and interests, is nevertheless inadequate as a guide to situations, such as, for example, embryo research and abortion where rights and interests conflict. This can best be brought out by returning to our example of the couple and the baby.

We have so far supposed that they gave no thought at all to the baby's rights and interests. But suppose that they did consider them only to dismiss them as, or even in the sincere conviction that they were, relatively unimportant. Could they then be described as having acknowledged the constraints that the baby's rights and interests set upon their conduct and thus be absolved of using her 'merely as a means'?[21] It would not ordinarily be supposed so. It would have to be shown that the couple were justified in dismissing the baby's claims.

Of course, no one would ordinarily demur at the claim that the couple's behaviour towards the baby was morally unjustified if the grounds remained as selfish and frivolous as earlier described. That situations are, however, rarely so morally unambiguous is apparent once we ask whether, to avoid using a person 'merely as a means', I must let her rights and interests prevail at any cost. Obviously not. For then I could be accused of failing to acknowledge the limits set upon my conduct by a second person's rights and interests which happen to conflict with those of the first.[22] Hence I could be accused of using her 'merely as a means'. If we are not to draw the conclusion – unpalatable to strict Kantians – that I cannot here avoid using someone 'merely as a means' and so must, in some circumstances, commit a wrong,[23] a criterion is required for the justifiable overriding of rights and interests. But Kant's second formulation of the categorical imperative, even as explicated, cannot itself supply the criterion.

We might try to supplement Kant's second formulation, by reference to his first formulation, of the categorical imperative: 'I ought never to act except in such a way that I can will that my maxim should become a universal law'.[24] But Kant believed that the two tests would lead independently to the same moral conclusions. Nevertheless the exceptionless moral precepts, supposedly yielded by the first formulation, do give a decisive answer in some cases where a reliance upon the second formulation will not. For instance, given that by the first criterion killing is exceptionlessly wrong, killing to save a life is wrong. Assuming that fetuses are persons, abortion is therefore immediately outlawed and the complicated balancing of rights and interests, required by the second formulation, rendered superfluous. But such crude certitude is only bought at the cost of suppressing the subtle and flexible responsiveness to individual situations that is now often regarded as indispensable to the proper resolution of moral dilemmas. Moreover, most people today would dismiss as far-fetched the idea that substantive moral precepts can be conjured out of a test of our rational consistency in willing that everyone follow them.[25]

Honed down to its essentials, Kant's prohibition on using

people 'merely as a means' is a claim about the constraints that one person's rights and interests lay upon other people's treatment of her. It cannot, as we have seen, tell us how to balance different people's rights and interests against each other. Nevertheless, it has a contemporary appeal lacked by Kant's first formulation of the categorical imperative, while its insistence on respect for human dignity is a safeguard against the excesses of utilitarianism. It seems quite clearly therefore to provide a sound starting-off point for the moral evaluation of our conduct even, as we have seen, towards those who are themselves incapable of desire or opinion.

*An attack on the consistency of (T)*

With Kant's notion of using people 'merely as means' clarified, I return to the original claim – that embryo research is never, whereas abortion is sometimes, morally permissible – to ask whether its consistency can be undermined by appeal to Kant's prohibition. I shall concentrate, as already noted, on Kennedy's version of the claim.

As we saw earlier, to undermine Kennedy's position it would be enough to show that the feature of embryo research which leads him to object to it is also exhibited by abortion. It could then be concluded that Kennedy is inconsistent in objecting to embryo research yet supporting abortion. On this issue, it is irrelevant whether possessing the feature in question renders either embryo research or abortion morally impermissible.

A more ambitious attack might, however, be mounted against Kennedy which attempts to demonstrate the stronger claim that if embryos are persons, then abortion is just as morally impermissible as embryo research since it too possesses the feature which leads Kennedy to condemn embryo research – namely, that the embryo is used 'merely as a means'. What follows is a composite argument I have gleaned from the literature.[26]

Kennedy's allegation that embryo research involves using an end in itself 'merely as a means' to an end, and is thus morally impermissible, may be conceded. For, if embryos are ends in themselves, then it is indeed morally impermissible to research upon them and then to kill them. But British abortion legislation permits killing the fetus to benefit others, though the fetus is an even more plausible candidate for the status of an end in itself, or person, than the fourteen day embryo. Consequently, for those, such as Kennedy, who claim that the embryo or fetus is an end in itself, abortion too (as currently permitted) involves using what is an end in itself 'merely as a means'. He cannot then consistently both object to embryo research and support abortion.

But this argument, though apparently cogent, is vague and elliptical. It is open to at least two interpretations, both of which are untenable.

On the first interpretation, its lynch pin is a persuasive redefinition of abortion as killing embryos and fetuses to benefit others. Once abortion is described as killing to benefit others we are apparently meant just to see that it involves using embryos and fetuses 'merely as means' and hence is, if embryos and fetuses are ends in themselves, morally impermissible. It would follow that we could not consistently allow abortion, yet ban embryo research, if the grounds for this latter prohibition are (as Kennedy makes clear) that it involves using what are ends in themselves 'merely as means'.

But we may object to the whole enterprise of persuasive redefinition as really just a covert way of expressing moral approval or disapproval. Merely to call abortion by derogatory names, even if that name is 'murder', will not settle its moral status. In fact, however, unlike the term 'murder', the phrase 'killing to benefit others' is so evaluatively ambiguous that we feel justified in allowing abortion to be thus characterised yet deny that it involves using the fetus 'merely as a means'. Moreover, if this evaluatively ambiguous phrase is used, then for the argument to be successful an account must be provided of why killing an embryo to benefit others is using it 'merely as a means'.

On the second interpretation, the argument might seem to offer just such an account. The characterisation of abortion as killing embryos and fetuses to benefit others is still crucial, but no longer gets us on its own to the conclusion that abortion involves using embryos and fetuses 'merely as means' and thus, if embryos and fetuses are ends in themselves, is morally impermissible. To reach this conclusion we must now first compare abortion, under the new description, with embryo research. The thought is: if researching upon, and then killing, embryos is using them 'merely as means', then so certainly is killing them to benefit others. Hence, if embryo research is morally objectionable so is abortion.

But this line of argument will only work if we are told just why researching on embryos, and then killing them, counts as using them 'merely as means'. For only then shall we be in a position to determine whether killing embryos and fetuses to benefit others also counts as such.

By now, however, it will have become apparent that what is really required, for the success of such an argument, is a common characterisation of abortion (as currently permitted) and embryo research that demonstrates that they both involve using embryos or fetuses 'merely as means'. To cling to the proposed characterisation of abortion as killing embryos and fetuses to benefit others, in an attempt to bring it into line with embryo research, only clouds the issue. I shall therefore put this move aside in the following discussion in which I apply the conclusions reached in my section on Kant.

It might be claimed that it is because they make use of the embryo that both embryo research and abortion (as currently permitted) involve using it 'merely as a means'. Certainly embryo research makes use of the embryo. For researchers, having facilitated its creation, either dissect it in order to gain new knowledge about disease, infertility and genetic abnormality or subject it to different culture mediums for information about the fluids most favourable for culturation of embryos *in vitro*.[27] Moreover, having used it in these ways, they are normally then obliged to destroy it, if it is not already dead.

But, by contrast, in simple abortion the embryo or fetus is neither killed to be (or in the process of being) made use of nor made use of and then killed, as in embryo research. It is, to invoke the distinction drawn earlier between someone's being a means and an obstacle to our ends, killed because it stands in the way of other people's ends. Moreover, no amount of talk about current abortion laws permitting the killing of embryos and fetuses for others' benefit will blur this distinction between abortion and these other procedures.

Secondly, again as Kant emphasised, for one person to use another 'merely as a means' it is not sufficient that he makes use of her. Hence it will not do in justification of the claim that embryo researchers use the embryo 'merely as a means' to cite the fact that the researcher makes use of the embryo, even though this use leads to its death. As we saw earlier, we must further show that, in making use of the embryo, with all the consequences this brings in its chain, she unjustifiably overrides the embryo's rights and interests. A similar demonstration would have to be made in the case of simple abortions. Making use of the embryo, even though this leads to its death, cannot then be the common description of embryo research and abortion which entails that both procedures involve using the embryo 'merely as a means'.

Alternatively, it might be pointed out that in both abortion and embryo research, killing the embryo or fetus is a means to some end (namely, benefiting others). Hence both involve using the embryo or fetus 'merely as a means'. But in embryo research it is not the killing of the embryo but the prior research which is a means to the end, for example, of benefiting others. However, with abortion, killing the fetus *is* the means to an end. But it does not in any case follow, as we again saw in our discussion of Kant, that because we perform an action as a means to an end that the person affected is used 'merely as a means'. Handing a cheque to the bank cashier as a means of drawing money out of the bank is not using her 'merely as a means' but only as a means. But can we kill someone as a means to an end without using her 'merely as a means'?

I cannot see, however, that it alters the moral status of killing, leaving aside the value of the ends, whether it is undertaken as a means to some end or is itself the end. My killing you is not better if I do it on an evil whim than if I do it to inherit your money. Either way, my action would, according to Kant's criteria, fall into the category of using you 'merely as a means'. On the other hand, some ends, as we shall see, may be considered to possess such overriding importance that an agent who kills as a means to achieving them is absolved of any charge of using the person he has killed 'merely as a means'.

Consider, for instance, the doctor faced with a situation in which a woman in labour will die if he does not crush the unborn child's skull. Here his killing the fetus is a means to an end but we may not conclude that he therefore uses the fetus 'merely as a means'. For an impressive case can be made out that the mother's right to life overrides the fetus's. (Incidentally, even accepting this defence of abortion, we might still describe the doctor as killing the fetus to benefit the mother provided our use of that term does not entail moral condemnation.) Embryo research and simple abortion, then, do not both involve killing as a means to an end. But, even if they did, it would not follow that they therefore involved using the embryo 'merely as a means'.

Now that we have dispersed some of the obfuscation associated with the evaluatively ambiguous expression killing to benefit others, we may reiterate the points which emerged from our discussion of Kant. To determine whether embryo research or abortion involves using the embryo or fetus, if it is a person, 'merely as a means', we must ask whether its rights are, in either instance, unjustifiably overriden. There is, however, no short cut to the answers. Merely gesturing towards the notion of use will not enable us to dispense with the painstaking balancing of rights and interests that the justification of both procedures demands. The contention that, if embryos and fetuses are persons, abortion as well as embryo research is morally impermissible, is hence still unsupported, and the attempt to demonstrate Kennedy's inconsistency, in objecting to embryo research yet supporting abortion, has failed.

## 2. New beginnings: satisfying the conditions for upholding (T)

*Justifying abortion if embryos and fetuses are persons*

As we have seen, Kennedy claims that embryo research is never, whereas abortion is sometimes, permissible on the grounds that embryo research, unlike abortion, always involves using the embyo 'merely as a means'. Now to demonstrate the consistency of this claim it is enough to show that there are putative justifications for abortion which are not available for embryo research.

However, consistency or inconsistency between moral

judgments does not settle the question of their validity since it only concerns the logical interrelationships between their justifications. Hence, to uphold Kennedy's position, these justifications have also to be defended. They must, in other words, be strong enough to absolve those who perform abortions of the charge of using the fetus, if it is a person, 'merely as a means'. In addition, it has to be shown that there are no independent, but equally powerful, justifications for the deaths of embryos involved in research. For, as we have noted, if there were, embryo research would sometimes be morally permissible which (T) denies.

If however we wished to uphold (T) categorically then we would also have to show either that embryos and fetuses are persons or that it is morally impermissible to use non-persons 'merely as a means'. I will consider the first two issues in this and the following section. The last issue, as I indicated earlier, would require extensive discussion for which there is no space here.

Consider, then, that apparently most compelling of justifications for abortion: saving the mother's life. Such a justification is obviously not available in the case of embryo research since the embryo, being *in vitro*, cannot endanger the mother. Therefore, if Kennedy were to hold that we may justifiably override the embryo's or fetus's right to life only when it puts the mother's life at risk, he would certainly be consistent. But is this justification valid if the fetus is a person?

The challenge is to show that there is a parallel between abortion, where the fetus poses a grievous threat to the mother's life, and other situations where it would be deemed morally acceptable to kill a person who threatens the life of others. Judith Jarvis Thompson, in a famous paper,[28] has likened abortion where the mother's life is at risk to killing in self-defence. But the fetus differs in two crucial respects from an ordinary assailant. It is dependent for survival upon the body of the person it is supposedly attacking and, secondly, since it is innocent of any intention to harm her, it can hardly be said to have 'forfeited' its right to life. A further objection is that the concept of self-defence is intolerably stretched by being made to cover cases where the victim does not strike back at her attacker in the heat of the moment, but coolly premeditates the killing and employs a third party to carry it out.

But, to take the first point, why should the fetus's depen-
dence upon her body for survival inhibit the mother from
defending her own life? If an assailant seizes me and places me
between himself and marksmen as a shield from bullets, he
needs my body to stay alive. But I am not therefore morally
debarred from throwing him off. Again, the mere absence of an
intention to harm on the part of the fetus is not an insuperable
obstacle to accepting Thompson's argument. For it would
hardly be reasonable to expect a woman not to defend herself
against a sleepwalker brandishing a knife because she knew he
had no intention to harm her.[29] Moreover, the idea is
increasingly being canvassed by philosophers that an individual may forfeit certain rights for harming another person even
unintentionally.[30]

Thompson herself has an answer[31] to the objection that it is
no part of the notion of self-defence that the business of
defence is given over to a third party and I shall not rehearse it
here. Suffice it to say that this objection would immediately
disintegrate if women were given the facilities to carry out their
own abortions, as is promised in America. The fairly recent
acquittal (1987) by an American court, on grounds of self-
defence, of a woman who contracted three men to kill her
violent husband shows that at least some courts are even
prepared to stretch the concept of self-defence to the extent
that the use of intermediary agents may be legally sanctioned.

The disanalogies between abortion and self-defence remain
striking enough to lead a few writers, in particular Roman
Catholics, to resist the claim that abortion may be justified to
save the mother's life. Nevertheless, once the three most
damaging objections are dealt with (and I hope my necessarily
brief remarks show that they are not insuperable), this
justification may well seem powerful enough to absolve those
who procure and perform abortions of using the fetus, even if it
is a person, 'merely as a means'.

Are the justifications for abortion countenanced by current
British legislation similarly powerful? Is damage to the
mother's health, short of a threat to her life, or psychological
damage either to her or to her other children sufficient to
override the fetus's right to life? These justifications for
abortion are not available in the case of embryo research, and
hence could serve as a basis for consistency in asserting (T). It is

doubtful however whether, if fetuses are persons, they are defensible.

Adopting Thompson's strategy, we may look for situations in which we would countenance killing an adult or child for the above reasons. But of course we shall find none. Indeed it is inconceivable that anyone would be acquitted of the murder of her ten-year-old child on grounds that he was affecting her health or psychologically damaging herself or her other children.

If, however, we turn from what I shall call 'the arguments from harm' to the women's rights argument (which again cannot be adduced to justify the destruction involved in embryo research), the case becomes proportionately stronger. It would also, unlike 'the arguments from harm', provide, as we shall see, a justification for abortion whenever the mother wants it and not merely when she has good moral reasons for wanting it.[32]

Women's rights supporters would argue that a woman, in seeking an abortion, cannot be compared with a woman intent on killing her child. Certainly both women are responsible either directly or indirectly for killing their offspring. However, the fetus, unlike the ten-year-old child, is using his unwilling mother's body to stay alive. Hence to uphold the ten-year-old's right to life against his murderous mother is only to maintain that he has a right not to be killed. But to uphold the fetus's right to life, though his mother wants an abortion, is to commit oneself, much more controversially, to the view that it has a right to continue to use her organs against her will.

But to allow the mother's right to determine what happens in and to her body to be overridden for the benefit of someone else is to use the mother herself 'merely as a means' and to deny her the very respect one wishes to accord the fetus. Moreover, such a lack of respect would be unthinkable in any situation other than pregnancy.

Consider, for instance, how morally disconcerted we would be if doctors were permitted to use a dead person's organs for transplantation, not merely without the dead person's consent, but even when he had expressly forbidden their use. Of course we acknowledge that, being dead, a person can suffer neither pain nor inconvenience by someone using his organs. Nor are they of any more use to him. Nevertheless, there is surely a general conviction that no one has a right to use his organs, unless the dead person has granted that right, even should other people desperately need them to stay alive.

To give one further example: even if a man needs a bone marrow transplant to survive, his sister, though she may be the only suitable donor, cannot be forced to help him. But then, the pro-abortionists will ask, is it not a moral outrage that a pregnant woman, especially if she has taken every precaution to avoid pregnancy (short of actually abstaining from intercourse), should unwillingly have to submit to someone else's use of her body? Thus the anti-abortionists' stress upon the separate personhood of the fetus is turned against them. It is, the pro-abortionists will finally allege, an indignity to ask a woman even to justify her wish to terminate her pregnancy.

Just as the parallel between abortion and the killing of the child fails in certain crucial respects, so too does the parallel between the woman wanting a termination and, for instance, the sister's refusal to donate bone marrow to her brother. For if we deny that the fetus has a right to use its mother's body against her will then, since the only way to rectify matters is to kill the fetus, we are endorsing a killing. But to deny the brother's right to his sister's bone marrow, since she does not wish to donate it, is only to condone her not helping him survive. To assert without further argument (and there is no space here to discuss the acts-omissions doctrine) that this distinction is irrelevant is to beg the question in favour of the right not to have one's body used against one's will over the prohibition on killing. We beg the question in the opposite direction, however, if we attempt to compare the wrongness of killing, for example, a trespasser in one's house with that of killing a fetus in one's womb. Women's rights proponents will object that someone who has an unwanted being lodged in her body is in a much more serious plight than someone who merely has a trespasser in her house and therefore is not subject to the same moral constraints.

One way out of this impasse is to deny that there is a head-on clash of principles at all since the pregnant woman's body is not really used against her will. Thus some writers claim that she has given a right to the fetus to use her body by the very act of intercourse. Others[33] more radically argue (mistakenly, I believe) that it is incoherent to speak of the fetus having no right to use the woman's body. We can, they hold, only be said to have no right to do something which we have an obligation not to do. But it would be absurd to maintain that the pre-embryo had an obligation not to implant in its mother's womb. The women's rights justification for abortion is not then conclusive. Its power, however, lies in the fact that it pits against the prohibition on killing a consideration which is not comparable with it: the right not to have one's body used against one's will. Different harms can, by contrast, be assessed on the same scale of values. Thus a justification for abortion in terms of, say, damage to the mother's health is immediately vulnerable to the objection that the harm to be avoided may be less than the harm to be inflicted.

Furthermore, in proportion to the relaxation of requirements as to how much harm to others the fetus must represent before it may be aborted, so the justifications for embryo research in terms of the benefits to be gained become increasingly compelling. If, for instance, we allow a woman to have an abortion to avoid tooth decay then it will be hard for us simultaneously to object to embryo research if, say, it is likely to result in the eradication of genetic abnormality. Our position, though remaining consistent, will gradually lose credibility until we are finally forced to admit that embryo research and abortion are either both morally permissible or both morally impermissible. The precise point at which even credibility in maintaining (T) is finally lost is hard to identify. Many would argue, however, that it has already been reached by current permissive interpretation of abortion legislation.

## Justifying embryo research if embryos are persons

The only decisively defensible justification for abortion if fetuses are persons is, I have suggested, threat to the mother's life. We have already demonstrated the consistency of maintaining (T) where this is regarded as the only circumstance which makes abortion morally permissible. But to validate this version of (T), we need to show not only, as we have sought to, that this justification is defensible but also that there are no independent but equally defensible justifications for embryo research. As already noted, however, embryo research can take place in two wholly different circumstances. This affects the kind and quality of justification that can be given and therefore requires comment.

Embryos may be deliberately created for research: for instance, when eggs donated by a woman during sterilisation are fertilised from a sperm bank. Here the expected benefits of research, such as the cure of infertility, the eradication of genetic abnormality and so on, must carry the burden of justifying not only the research itself but also the deliberate creation of embryos to be destroyed in the process of being used to benefit others.

The embryos on which it is proposed to research may however be those left over after the process of IVF. Now if, as many maintain, it is necessary to fertilise more than one of a woman's eggs if she is to have even a small chance of becoming pregnant, then the benefits of IVF must bear the weight of justifying the creation of embryos, subsequently to be destroyed. In other words, it is the benefit to an infertile couple of having children that has here to be balanced against the harm suffered by the spare embryos.

Let us suppose that benefit to an infertile couple were a defensible justification for wastage of spare embryos, and thus for IVF as currently practised. It would not automatically follow that research on these embryos was also justified. However, a new kind of justification for the latter would now become possible. For the wastage of spare embryos could be regarded as a 'necessary evil' from which we should salvage whatever good we could. But no such appeal can be made in the case of research upon embryos deliberately created for the purpose of research.

Indeed it is difficult to see how, if embryos are persons, the benefits of research, however great, could ever justify creating them for this purpose. It would, after all, be unthinkable that a child be brought into the world to be destroyed in the process of being researched upon, even if a cure for cancer resulted. The claim that embryo research is never permissible whereas abortion is permissible if the pregnancy threatens the mother's life will hardly then be undermined from this quarter.

But might not research upon the spare embryos of IVF be defensible if their death is construed as a 'necessary evil' from which we should try to salvage what good we can? Even here, however, we should not be over-impressed by the fact that the death of spare embryos is inevitable, assuming that freezing is undesirable and the chances are minimal of finding a woman willing to have a rejected embryo implanted into her. It would, after all, be inconceivable that even the most painless research, whatever its benefits to humanity, should be allowed upon a child or adult just because she was terminally ill. Even research after death would require, as we have seen, some kind of consent.

This type of justification for research will in any case only be coherent if IVF has been shown to have such beneficial results that it is imperative, despite the toll in embryo lives, that it be available to infertile couples. But the proponents of IVF can only set against the certain destruction of hundreds of spare embryos, and of all those embryos which are implanted unsuccessfully, the benefit for a few lucky infertile couples of having a child. Some practitioners of IVF even maintain that its low success rate and subsequent toll in embryo lives makes it imperative that the government either fund research for improving the techniques or prohibit it altogether.[34]

I conclude then that, if embryos and fetuses are persons, (T) may be decisively upheld when the circumstances that make abortion morally permissible are restricted to threat to the mother's life. If the womens' rights arguments were however to be endorsed, we could conclude, more strongly than (T), that embryo research is never, but abortion is always, morally permissible when the mother wants it.[35]

## 3. Abortion is immoral, and hence never permissible, but embryo research and fetal transplantation are more immoral

Suppose someone insists that, despite the above considerations, even if a fetus endangers its mother's life, its own right to life cannot be justifiably overridden. But embryo researchers and surgeons who perform fetal transplantation not only use embryos and fetuses 'merely as means' (as does abortion) but also make use of them. They thus also exploit the embryos and fetuses and their activities are even more immoral than abortion.

Such a position, of course, betrays once again, though now

dressed up in the emotive language of exploitation, the superstition that injuring someone in the course of making use of her is worse than injuring her because she is an obstacle to one's ends. But we are asked here to assent to a general distinction between the two types of action not, as before, in terms of the latter being moral but the former being immoral, but in terms of the two possessing different degrees of immorality. Is such a position tenable?

We earlier distinguished between two ways in which we may use someone 'merely as a means', depending upon whether she is a means or an obstacle to our ends. If we reserve the term 'exploitation', as seems appropriate, for using someone merely as a means in the first sense, then we can contrast exploiting someone with other ways of using her 'merely as a means'.

The distinction may be illustrated by our example of the couple and the baby. If the couple return her to the adoption agency because keeping her would demand some small financial sacrifice, then they have used her 'merely as a means' in the second sense. For all that counts with them is that she stands in the way of their getting what they want. Were they, however, to be able to rid themselves of the child by, say, selling her, then they would be using her 'merely as a means' in the first sense too, and thus exploiting her. For they would then make getting rid of her actually pay.

But is exploitation an evil over and above using someone 'merely as a means'? Now admittedly selling the baby seems to compound the evil of just getting rid of her. But it is not, I believe, a worse wrong. Indeed, if it is equally wrong, this is due, I suggest, not to its character as exploitation but to a merely contingent feature of this particular exploitation. This becomes apparent once we recognise, for instance, that killing a fetus because it is an obstacle to accomplishing our ends can sometimes be more morally repugnant than killing it as a means to our accomplishing them, though only in the latter instance do we actually exploit it. A European socialite who, in order not to miss a skiing holiday, has a 28-week abortion may well seem more morally reprehensible than a third world woman who, on pain of starving to death, has her fetus aborted and sells its brain tissue. Again, an actress who has an abortion because she thinks pregnancy will spoil her figure seems more morally culpable than the altruistic woman who deliberately becomes pregnant and has an abortion so that she can donate its brain tissue for the cure of Parkinsonism.

To return to our original couple, if selling the baby, and thus exploiting her, seems as much of a wrong as just callously returning her to the agency, it is because the same unedifying selfishness and self-seeking permeate both actions. But then exploitation (especially when it is understood broadly enough to accommodate cases where the motive is not narrowly selfish) is in itself no more wrong than other ways of using someone 'merely as a means'.

Why should people suppose otherwise? They are impressed, I suspect, by the fact that we typically exploit a person for gain and, hence, cannot offer as an excuse for our ill-treating her that she was, even minimally, damaging to our or others' interests. This strikes them with particular force when they reflect upon embryo research and fetal transplantation, where the embryo or fetus is patently of no harm to anyone. Observing that there is no connection at all between the existence of the unfortunate embryo and the diseases which strike people down and for which embryo researchers and fetal transplant surgeons hope to find a cure, they are led to condemn these procedures even more strongly than abortion.

Nevertheless, it cannot be the mere absence of a causal link between the victim of exploitation and some undesirable situation which her exploiter wishes to prevent which accounts for the peculiar wrongness of exploitation, for such a link is absent when we, quite acceptably, make use of someone. Nor, as our examples show, does the absence of this link make exploitation specially pernicious among the ways of using someone 'merely as a means'.

Indeed it is hard to see how the absence of such a link could render an otherwise moral action immoral (or make an already immoral action more immoral) when its presence cannot turn an otherwise immoral action into a moral one. Yet, as we have seen, an abortion does not become morally right just by virtue of the fact that, being pregnant, a woman is prevented from taking the skiing holiday she desires. (Indeed some writers, such as Finnis, a supporter of the doctrine of double effect, far from regarding the presence of this link as even necessary if abortion is to be morally permissible, hold, mistakenly I believe, that it is sufficient for an abortion's moral impermissibility.[36])

But the distinction between embryo research and fetal transplantation on the one hand and abortion on the other, is not in any case coextensive with that between killing the embryo or fetus to make use of it (where the link is absent) and killing it because its existence impedes other people's ends; for abortion could be undertaken to obtain fetal brain tissue for transplantation (although the BMA has declared such an action 'utterly repugnant').

I have not so far mentioned those situations where the fetus, through no intention of the transplant surgeon, is already dead when it arrives on the operating table and where consequently talk of exploitation is possibly inappropriate. I turn, however, to the moral propriety of salvaging good from evil in the next section.

## 4. Immoral actions that have a potential for good: the problem posed by fetal transplantation for those who believe abortion immoral: two positions

*Nothing evil can be made good by its consequences*

If abortion *were* an evil (as many people fervently believe) the question would arise as to what to make of the above claims, so frequently and stridently voiced in relation to fetal transplantation.

To hold that nothing evil can be made good by its consequences is to occupy a midway position between the utilitarians and those who declare pessimistically that 'no good can come of evil'. For utilitarians an abortion, the immediate consequences of which produce a net harm, may in the end prove to have been a good. It will all depend upon whether we can turn these consequences to advantage in producing benefits that outweigh the original harm.

But those who maintain that 'nothing evil can be made good by its consequences' disagree. If abortion is an evil then, for these 'moderates' (as I shall call them), it cannot be transformed into a good, however great are the benefits that may ultimately be derived from it. The moral character of an action is, so to speak, fixed. Nevertheless, their position does not commit them to prohibiting people from taking advantage of the consequences of an evil action. They deny only that an evil action can itself be made good by its consequences, not that good can be salvaged from evil.

A criterion will be required, however, to distinguish between salvaging good from evil and actually condoning evil. The criterion that most obviously suggests itself is whether or not the person, who now wishes to take advantage of the consequences of an evil action, could have prevented or tried to prevent it. If she could not have prevented it then taking advantage of its consequences will only result in salvaging good from evil. If she could have prevented it, but chose not to, she will be condoning evil. By this criterion, a doctor who transplants the heart and lungs of the victim of a murder, which she did not know was taking place, will not lay herself open to the charge of condoning evil.

But suppose our 'moderates' regard abortion as morally impermissible, although it is legal. Would the above criterion also enable them to determine what their attitude should be to a doctor who takes advantage of legalised abortions to perform fetal transplants? But the criterion is much less helpful than in the murder situation. With murder, an illegal act, the doctor's situation is unambiguous: if she did not know it was being committed, at the time it was being committed, then she had no chance of preventing it. But with legalised abortion the situation is different. The doctor may not have known that this particular abortion was taking place but she will know that abortions are being performed. Again, even if she had known about this particular abortion and could not have done anything to stop it, she could be fighting for reform of the law.

Matters are still further complicated by her own moral attitude to abortion. Consequently, there are three possible scenarios:

1. She performs fetal transplants, fully approving the abortions which make them possible and therefore doing nothing to get the law repealed.

2. She performs fetal transplants; but though she shares the moderates' abhorrence of abortion, does nothing to get the law repealed.

3. She performs fetal transplants, though she both shares the moderates' abhorrence of abortion and agitates to get the law repealed.

With the first scenario, the 'moderates' have the option, if they condemn her for condoning evil, of excusing her on the grounds that her action, though in accordance with her own moral principles, is misguided. However, as I have already indicated, the criterion does not determine whether they should condemn her in the first place.

Turning to the second scenario, it may perhaps help to observe that an almost analogous dilemma could arise with regard to capital punishment. Would it, for instance, be right for a doctor, morally opposed to capital punishment, to use the kidney of a person hanged for murder to save someone's life? Of course, in some respects, this situation could prove even more morally perplexing than fetal transplantation. For the executed man may have given consent for his kidney to be used. If consent, however, were given by the dead man's relatives, then a parallel would be restored with fetal transplantation which requires consent by the aborted fetus's mother. Again, we may speculate here as to whether our answer would be different if we knew that the doctor was agitating for reform of the law allowing capital punishment.

Of course, 'moderates', opposed to abortion, might wish to prohibit even those who could not have prevented an abortion from taking advantage of its consequences. They may refrain from accusing such people of *condoning* evil, yet argue that the good that is seen to result from using fetal brain tissue to cure Parkinsonism might lead to the false conclusion that abortion is less bad than it really is. This fear evidently underlies the often voiced imperative that we must not let a situation arise where a woman can be swayed in her decision to have an abortion by the consideration that it will not only be a solution to her own personal difficulties but also of benefit to others. She must not, in other words, be allowed to salve her conscience by offering her aborted fetus's brain tissue for use in transplantation.

## No good can come of evil

I turn finally to the deeply pessimistic conviction that no good can come of evil. To be committed to such a view is to hold uncompromisingly that the evil character of an evil action extends to every one of its consequences, whether intended or unintended by the agent. Any apparent good that is derived from them is, it is believed, wholly illusory. Moreover, to try to take advantage of the consequences is to become, if not an instrument of evil then certainly embroiled in and contaminated by evil. If we are inclined to dismiss these views as over-dramatic, even hysterical, it is important to emphasise that many of us experience their power when we reflect upon what our attitude should be to atrocities. Suppose, for instance, it were to come to light that mutilating medical experiments, performed by Nazis upon Jewish inmates of concentration camps during the last war, resulted in a cure for cancer. The relevant documents, we learn, are stored away under lock and key in Zürich. Would it be unreasonable for the Israeli government, in the name of those dead Jews, to demand that we, though unborn when these crimes were committed, tear up the papers and forgo the fruits of knowledge acquired at the price of such suffering and death?

Now if we morally object to abortion yet are inclined to countenance fetal transplantation, pending reform of the abortion laws, this may not be because we are 'moderates' but rather because we do not regard the killing of an embryo or fetus as sufficiently atrocious. But the pro-life lobby would have us believe that it is an atrocity on a par with the Nazis' extermination of the Jews. It is a matter of urgency then to decide exactly where we stand on this issue. I hope the foregoing may help to sort out the surrounding confusions.[37]

Notes and references

1 Research which is not designed to facilitate the replacement of embryos into the womb – henceforth referred to as embryo research.

2 Henceforth referred to as fetal transplantation.

3 It is usually assumed that a fetus may (for the reasons permitted) lawfully be aborted up to 28 weeks. But, as Professor Ian Kennedy in Treat me right (Oxford, Clarendon Press, 1988, pages 48–51) pointed out, to abort a viable fetus even before 28 weeks contravenes the Infant Life (Preservation) Act of 1929 which forbids the destruction of any child 'capable of being born alive'.

4 The Abortion Act, 1967.

5 These relatively moderate positions would seem, as Michael
Lockwood suggested to me, to reflect the belief that creating an
embryo for experimentation, or aborting a fetus in order to
transplant tissue, contravenes the principle of double effect in a
way that using the 'spare' embryos of IVF or fetuses aborted for
reasons unconnected with transplantation does not. This rationale
is made explicit in the Warnock report (Department of Health
and Social Security. Report of the Committee of Inquiry into
Human Fertilisation and Embryology. Cmnd 9314 (Chairman:
Dame Mary Warnock) London, HMSO, 1984, pages 66–69).

6 See Jeremy Brown. Research on human embryos – a justification.
Journal of Medical Ethics, 12, 4, December 1986, pages 201–205.

7 Ian Kennedy. Let the law take on the test tube. The Times,
26 May 1984.

8 Professor Ian Kennedy in The Times article (see 7 above) states
unequivocally that embryo research using embryos specially
created for that purpose is always morally impermissible. There is
some dispute however about his views concerning research upon
the spare embryos of IVF. I take his position to be as follows: if
the creation of excess embryos during IVF were morally justified,
then we might take advantage of their existence for research; but
spare embryos are often created purely for research and therefore
research upon them is morally impermissible; in any case even if
their creation did improve the chances of a successful implanta-
tion, this would not render it morally justifiable and therefore
research using spare embryos would remain morally impermissible.
Hence, it seems evident that he is, in effect, opposed to all embryo
research.

9 But see 8 above.

10 Unless otherwise stated the word abortion in the text always
refers to abortion on the grounds currently permitted and where
fetal material is not used for transplantation.

11 'Act in such a way that you always treat humanity, whether in
your own person or in the person of any other, never merely as a
means, but always at the same time as an end' (see 14 below).

12 Henceforth I shall always refer to Kennedy's version of (T).

13 See, for instance, Keith Ward's excellent discussion in Persons,
kinds and capacities. In: Peter Byrne (ed). Rights and wrongs in

medicine: King's College Studies 1985–6. London King Edward's Hospital Fund for London, 1986, pages 53–79.

14 Immanuel Kant. Groundwork of the metaphysic of morals (second edition). In: H J Paton (translator). Moral Law, Hutchinson, 1972.

15 See 14 above, page 91.

16 See, for instance, D D Raphael. Moral philosophy, Oxford, Oxford University Press, 1984, pages 56–57; Richard Norman. The moral philosophers: an introduction to ethics. Oxford, Oxford University Press, 1985, page 118.

17 See 14 above, page 92.

18 See 14 above, page 90.

19 We might add here 'or unlike couples who use, as methods of contraception, the intra-uterine device or post-coital pill'. Peter Byrne drew my attention to this extension of my claim.

20 My claim here, as Jonathan Barnes pointed out to me, could be strengthened. For it is not only that harming someone is not intrinsic to using someone 'merely as a means' (as here interpreted) but that benefiting someone does not ensure that she is not used 'merely as a means'. Indeed, I may benefit someone by using her 'merely as a means' or even use her 'merely as a means' in order to benefit her. Thus, a doctor may be accused of using her patient 'merely as a means' when she denies him, in what she believes to be his own good, knowledge he requires to make informed consent to a proposed medical treatment.

21 This question was originally suggested to me by Kenneth Campbell.

22 A point well made by C D Broad in Five types of ethical theory. London, Kegan Paul, 1930, page 132.

23 Some writers (see particularly B Williams. Moral luck. Cambridge, Cambridge University Press, 1981, pages 20–39) now maintain, in opposition to Kant, that even in situations where we had no choice but to act as we did or where luck played a role, we may be held morally responsible for the outcome. I discuss this idea in my article, Precarious virtue. Phronesis, XXII, 1, 1987, pages 101–131.

24 See 14 above, page 67.

25  For a different interpretation of Kant's first formulation see
    R Green. Religious reason. Oxford, Oxford University Press,
    1978.

26  But I draw chiefly upon Jeremy Brown, see 6 above.

27  See Mary J Seller and Elliot Philipp. Reasons for wishing to
    perform research on human embryos. In: G R Dunstan and M J
    Seller (eds). The status of the human embryo: perspectives from
    moral tradition. London, King Edward's Hospital Fund for
    London, 1988, pages 22–32.

28  Judith J Thompson. A defence of abortion. In: Ronald M
    Dworkin (ed). The philosophy of law. Oxford, Oxford University
    Press, 1977, pages 112–128.

29  I am indebted to Julie Stone for this example.

30  See, for instance, Vinit Haksar. Excuses and voluntary conduct.
    Ethics, January 1986. Haksar, though prepared to countenance
    punishing a person for unintentionally harming another, does not
    wish, like Williams (see 23 above), to hold her morally respon-
    sible for, or guilty of, wrong doing. But I have argued elsewhere
    (Acceptance and morality. Philosophy, 58, 1983, pages 433–453)
    that the notion of punishment cannot coherently be divorced
    from the ideas of moral responsibility and guilt.

31  See 28 above, page 116.

32  Jonathan Barnes suggested to me that any credible defence of
    abortion requires that the woman has good moral reasons for
    wanting an abortion. Women's rights proponents of abortion,
    however, regarding such a requirement as an insult to a woman's
    dignity and a violation of her autonomy, stipulate that there be
    no restrictions whatsoever on abortion. See, for instance, the
    National Abortion Campaign's pamphlet, Abortion: our struggle
    for control, page 18.

33  J Finnis. The rights and wrongs of abortion. In: Ronald M
    Dworkin (ed). The philosophy of law. Oxford, Oxford University
    Press, 1977, pages 129–152.

34  This point was put forcibly to me by Dr John Parsons of the IVF
    unit at King's College Hospital.

35  This qualification (for which I am indebted to Jonathan Barnes) is
    not trivial, for abortion would not be permissible where the
    father, but not the mother, wanted it.

36 See 33 above, page 142. Finnis argues that if it were the existence of the fetus itself that were endangering the mother's life as opposed, for example, to her having a cancerous womb then, in aborting it, the doctor would be deliberately aiming at its death which is morally impermissible.

37 Apart from those mentioned above, I am also indebted to Professor Ian Kennedy and to A R Jonckheere for reading and commenting on an earlier draft of this chapter.

# Can medical ethics be taught?

Roger Higgs

A Peanuts cartoon of a decade ago hangs like the sword of
Damocles over my desk. Lucy holds up her hand in class. 'You
know what Oscar Wilde said, Ma'am? He said, "Nothing that
is worth knowing can be taught". Nothing personal, Ma'am
...' If we do think that the application of ethical thinking
to health care is important, there is a challenge here that is
worth taking up. What is there about medical ethics that makes
us ask the question? If Latin, Lithuanian, macro-economics or
mediaeval ecclesiology are on the curriculum, why not medical
ethics? Is there something special about the problems which
this discipline addresses, and therefore perhaps something
different about the type of teaching which needs to be used?

The questions which medical ethics address ultimately
derive, both historically and academically, from clinical practice – that is, the pursuit or delivery of health care. (I shall use
'medical ethics' in a rather old-fashioned way, to indicate the
area of interest of anyone who is involved in the delivery or
receipt of health care and not just, as is often used nowadays, to
indicate the specific concern of doctors.) That is not to say that
if clinical practice were to change, medical ethics would
become irrelevant: even 'health for all' raises enough issues to
be getting on with. Rather, it is to remind ourselves that if ideas
emerge for study, they will always have to be tested in action,
and that medical activities in turn require an examination of the
ideas that lie behind them. Medical ethics gets put to use. It is
not an armchair subject, although it is possibly now a
commonroom or cafeteria one. The effects of this involvement
with practice have been dramatic both upon medicine and
upon ethics. Words such as 'autonomy', foreign to ward
rounds or surgeries in the past, are now regularly part of

clinical discussion, and the introduction to a recent BBC series on philosophy suggested that a recent revival of interest in the study of practical ethics among philosophers had been created by the needs of medical ethics.[1] In some countries philosophers and moralists have been involved in a direct way in clinical decisions. But whatever system might be introduced, research and thinking in medical ethics is tested in the laboratory of practice, whether that is personal, managerial, epidemiological or professional practice, and whatever point of the health care system may be under examination.

This claim, obvious to some, should not be read as undervaluing those who do not work in clinical practice, or of challenging the value of abstract thinking in general.[2] It is not an argument for crude pragmatism, and certainly not for a doctrinaire approach or for idealism. Nor am I trying to raise the status of medical ethics by association, or claim some extra utility. We have been warned, correctly, not to expect too much from our studies.[3] In clinical practice the rush and bustle, pressure on time and funds, the need for a positive outcome, the volume of possible work and the strong emotions attached to success or failure may all militate against clear thinking. Nevertheless, in whatever way we take 'time off' to do this necessary thinking, that thinking must remain in dialogue with practice. The close association between doing and thinking may well make both activities more arduous and may also make medical ethics mucky, exasperating, or even, in intolerant times, dangerous. But if it won't work, it won't wash.

Thus, I modify the question. Can the *practice* of medical ethics be taught, or even (which is a different question), can medical ethics be taught *in practice*? Consider an example from a recent multiprofessional discussion at a local psychiatric hospital. Miss JA, a young woman of 21 who was severely mentally handicapped, became pregnant by a man who then deserted her. At an antenatal clinic attendance she became psychiatrically disturbed and was admitted to a mental hospital ward for assessment. Although she had lived up until then with her parents, on the ward she made a series of statements which suggested that she had been sexually abused by her father in the past, and other evidence subsequently obtained appeared to support this. She was retained on the ward and the placing of the new mother and baby thus became a major concern. Her parents were keen to have them in their home, and Miss JA was very keen to go. But because the new baby was a girl, the allegations against the grandfather made returning them both to his home a difficult option. Miss JA still required help with household and mothering tasks but refused to go into a supervised hostel. Adoption had been raised with her, but it was thought that she didn't understand this well and was likely to react very badly to separation from her new baby.

At the discussion it was pointed out that a decision was urgently needed, because of issues of bonding in both directions and for the sake of the baby's development. The debate was important because of its multidisciplinary nature, and uncomfortable because of the need to make proxy decisions based on very little personal knowledge and few clinical or scientific guidelines. It was likely that the future was clouded, in whichever way it was viewed. Returning the child to live with a known child abuser seemed impossible, although this accusation could not be formally proved. The mother had still to have help with most daily activities for herself and the child, although there were some who felt that this potential had not been fully explored. Removing the child from the mother, if the care were to be institutional, might not provide well for the child and was certain to make the mother and grandparents extremely upset at the very least. The possibility that the mother would become pregnant again to fill the gap that was left, or simply pick up her baby and walk off, made it hard to escape from a consequentialist style of thinking. Yet a decision had to be made.

This case will be discussed in detail elsewhere. But it is instructive because through it we may focus on some of the issues which make ethical analysis in health care so vital but so hard to do (and so often hard to teach). It is also instructive because it brings us face to face with some of the ways in which clinical practice itself is problematic. Outsiders may be surprised to learn that there is often an uneasy relationship between clinical practice and the teaching which most practitioners received before qualification. It is not long after finals, and certainly by the time that doctors or nurses come into community practice, that they realise that many of the solutions and even the structures given to the problems which they were taught in their medical or nursing schools now no longer seem satisfactory or easily applicable. In the setting of a large teaching institution, many human problems that face professionals in clinical work are made manageable by forcing them into a particular medical framework and applying medical rules. This may sometimes be helpful in reaching a form of solution, and gives a structure which is known and tested and can be depended upon. But imposing a structure upon something implies an element of distortion: putting a limiting frame around a problem suggests that something may well be left out. If the man who has had his heart attack is under emotional pressure and smokes heavily in order to cope, simple medical solutions may not be appropriate or sufficient. In Miss JA's case, the medical model could be argued to be totally inappropriate; and yet she is there in medical care. And something has to be done.

At this point it may be a relief to discover that professionals of all types commonly find that the precepts which they were given in their training do not pass the test of practice. Donald Schön expresses it graphically in *Educating the Reflective Practitioner* when he introduces the scene. 'In the varied topography of professional practice, there is a high, hard ground overlooking a swamp. On the high ground, manageable problems lend themselves to solution through the application of research-based theory and technique. In the swampy lowland, messy, confusing problems defy technical solution. The irony of this situation is that ... in the swamp lie the problems of greatest human concern.'[4] There are few practising professionals for whom this will not ring loud bells. It is the dilemma of rigor versus relevance. Even if a technical rational solution is immediately helpful in the context of practice, before this can be applied the problem still has to be constructed. Practitioners have an ontological task and are, in Nelson Goodman's phrase, world makers, creating sense and direction for themselves and their clients.[5]

This process may create structures which look very different from those of the teaching institution, and may express themselves in a multitude of different ways. To return to our example of Miss JA: is she a product of society's lack of care, or part of the spectrum of genetic disorder? Does the solution lie in more effective social support, or in a change in economic priorities? Is it an issue of more detailed psychological assessment, or of more research into the effects of care? Could better education for the mentally handicapped have provided an answer? Is she a not very bright girl who needs a lot of love and attention? Is it a question of parental rights versus children's welfare? These are but a few of the ways in which an analysis could lead. But some important points emerge from this view of professional practice. One is that most thoughtful practitioners must live and work with a large measure of uncertainty, whatever their specialism or expertise. The task is to name and to frame, but, as we have seen, certainty can only be achieved at a price. The practitioner therefore has to acquire and develop judgment to cope with the many unknown as well as the known factors, and to look for guidelines where and when she can while distorting as little as possible. So, while searching for universal or at least generally valid ideas, the practitioner holds in mind the uniqueness of each case. If this process is to be successful, conflicts between values have to be acknowledged and brought out rather than suppressed. The more one looks, the more such conflicts are seen to be at the heart, and not on the fringe, of good professional work. Since medical ethics has much to offer in a debate about values, this analysis defies us to find a case which does *not* have an ethical component.

This conclusion may not be extraordinary to those working in medical ethics, but it may not be the way in which practitioners normally view their own work. Although the patient rather than the clinical task is increasingly seen as the focus of medical activity, medical ethics may ask the practitioner to think again about the identification of the 'patient'. In the discussion about Miss JA, should the focus be on the mother, the baby, the original family, or the person who decided to admit a pregnant woman with mental handicap to a psychiatric hospital in the first place? The 'patient' could be seen as the psychiatric or social service support team, or even the society which allows such a dilemma to arise. This line of analysis also may raise the question of the limit of professional expertise. It is not uncommon in discussion of cases such as that of Miss JA to hear at some stage a statement to the effect that things would be different if the patient were not making an irrational judgment, assumption or request. The expropriation of reasoning and rationality by professionals (even professionals in medical ethics) may be an attempt to rise above the swamp, but it is a move which we should treat with suspicion. The psychologist may be an expert in assessing mental capacity, but Miss JA, however inarticulate she may be, has expert knowledge of her own experiences and has her own line of reasoning. This cannot be ignored. Thus the expertise of the psychologist in assessing and predicting must be laid alongside the expertise of Miss JA in her own history. If this is hard to reach or difficult for the professional to comprehend, the search is on for more skill to enable others to understand what she has to say, even if this is not or cannot be the final arbiter. Professional practice in the swamp must face up to the necessity of sharing expertise and decision-making with those properly involved. This is well expressed in the title and substance of the publication by David Tuckett and his colleagues, *Meetings Between Experts.*[6]

Medical ethics has been at the forefront of some of this discussion by giving pride of place to respect for autonomy as an important guideline balanced with the other principles (as outlined in Raanan Gillon's work).[7] We have described additional work that may need to be done to bridge the gap that may still be left between these principles and the case or situation under examination, especially where competence is in doubt or choice is being deliberately, but perhaps inappropriately, delegated.[8]

Consideration of these issues may lead practitioners towards collecting different sets of data from those suggested to them by their original clinical teachers, and to do this may need new skills. These may include the ability to empathise, to consider personal rather than public histories, and to focus on potential more than pathology. A multidimensional ethical assessment cannot be made without considering the problem from all possible perspectives. But if medical art is long, life is short and to a hard-pressed professional these ideas may come as yet another unwelcome burden. If we are convinced that clinical ethics is part and parcel of clinical practice, how can we prepare ourselves and our colleagues to work in this way? Can it be taught?

We should have no difficulty in teaching or learning about the concepts. Clear thinking should have no opponents at any level, but how can these concepts be brought into practice?

Here we should examine our educational task. We are not talking about pedagogy, the instruction of children, but about the instruction of adult men and women called in educational jargon (with scant regard to gender and classical Greek usage) *androgogy*. The effectiveness of teaching in this sphere can only be evaluated by seeing some change in behaviour among the learners. Many studies bear witness to the strange way in which the effects teachers have on learners are unstable.[9] Learner outcomes are often unrelated to teacher behaviour. The teacher may teach, but what the learner learns may be quite different. The situation is summarised by Brundage and MacKeracher thus: 'The best predictor we have is that ... behaviour is a function of the interaction between person and environment ... a teacher must be considered as an influential part of a learner's environment through the provision of guidance, structure, information, feedback, reinforcement, and support.' But it is the learner who learns. Adults, unlike children, may bring many important life experiences to their learning which may block or impede their study. Learning needs are related to current life situations and the curriculum should be planned in a way which allows an adult learner to negotiate and design his or her own learning programme. Adult learners are independent, but they are responsible and expected to be productive. They bring well-formed attitudes, self-esteem, motivation, perceptions and emotions to 'school'. If these are not acknowledged and catered for, learning will not take place. If it doesn't click, it won't stick.[10]

These ideas come into sharp relief when the need is to learn about medical ethics. Many of the ways in which adult learners have come to structure ideas may be in conflict with the new concepts, and there may be, as we have seen, a feeling that 'it cannot work' or 'there just isn't time'. While constructing or reconstructing a problem, the learner must engage with it, must take it on board as a real problem – that is, one that makes sense and presents real issues to him or her. If the people with whom professionals are asked to consider themselves engaged feel alien in some sense, this feeling has to be overcome. Most young professionals lack first-hand experience of major illness, racial discrimination, or poverty, and all can be assumed to have no first-hand experience at all of mental handicap or of old age. So the construction must spread by extending the meanings, values, skills and strategies which have been acquired from previous experience. This may be more extensive than the teacher imagines. Undergraduate students often have more personal experience of death than is expected: the tragedy of road accidents and HIV infection means that not a few young professionals may now have lost friends or acquaintances of their own age. Many of us have elderly relatives, and can remember clearly, if we try, what it was like as a child to be patronised. If the environment for discussion is made to feel safe, experiences of despair or disorientation may be shared in a group. Professional and personal development may have been made at some loss, and in different ways by men and women.[11] This concept of education, however, brings us back to two ideas expressed in antiquity: that of the importance of knowing yourself and, as expressed in Plato's *Meno*, that of education as a rediscovery of things that had already been learnt.

Using these methods in undergraduate and postgraduate education in general practice studies, we have seen changes which convince that medical ethics has been learnt. In some sense we cannot avoid learning by doing, even if in simulated practice. However, time must be made in all professional practice and at all stages for reflection and discussion. Medical ethics cannot be applied, any more than any of the other 'basic' sciences or fields of knowledge, as a remedial activity tacked on to the end of the curriculum, or offered as an optional extra for those going for honours or destined for community practice. The dialogue between rigour and relevance must be established and become a lifetime occupation. Medical ethics may not be as easy as we think to teach, but it can and must be learnt. But without the regular chance to examine oneself, to challenge routines and to make the learning personally relevant, I do not think important learning in the field of clinical ethics will take place.

Notes and references

1 Introduction to the Great Philosophers series, Bryan Magee, transmitted in 1987 by the BBC.

2 Onora O'Neill. What's so wrong about being abstract. Cognito, Summer 1987.

3  R S Downie and Elizabeth Telfer. Caring and curing: a philosophy of medicine and social work. London, Methuen, 1980, pages 1–5.

4  Donald A Schön. Educating the reflective practitioner. San Francisco, Jossey-Bass, 1987.

5  Nelson Goodman. Ways of world making. Indianapolis, Hackett, 1978.

6  David Tucket and others. Meetings between experts: an approach to sharing ideas in medical consultations. London, Tavistock Publications, 1985.

7  Raanan Gillon. Philosophical medical ethics. In: This book or else ... London, John Wiley, 1986.

8  Alastair V Campbell and Roger Higgs. In that case: medical ethics in everyday practice. London, Darton, Longman and Todd in association with the Journal of Medical Ethics, 1982.

9  D D Pratt. Instructor behaviour and psychological climate in adult learning. Paper presented to the Adult Education Research Conference, Ann Arbor, Michigan, 1979.

10  Donald Brundage and Dorothy MacKeracher. Adult learning principles and the application to program planning. Ontario, Ministry of Education, 1980.

11  Carol Gilligan. In a different voice. Harvard University Press, 1982.

# Teaching medical ethics: impressions from the USA

Raanan Gillon

In the spring of 1984 I was able to spend six weeks visiting medical ethics teaching establishments in the USA.* Given the current interest in teaching medical ethics now evident in Britain, the rest of Europe and the Commonwealth, it may be worth resurrecting some of the information and impressions I garnered during that visit, outlining some of the ways medical ethics is being taught in the States and my doubtless idiosyncratic assessment of what we in Britain might learn from the American experience.

## Two concepts of medical ethics

It is perhaps worth distinguishing at the outset two different concepts of medical ethics and of medical ethics education. In one sense, doctors have been receiving medical ethics education at least since the time of Hippocrates. Thus the medical profession has accepted the moral principles underlying the Hippocratic Oath and/or its modern variants and developments for the last 2500 years, and it educates its members to conform to the precepts of these ethical codes and ensures their compliance. The most important components of such education are probably 'socialisation' and 'role modelling'. Powerful psychosocial pressures are brought to bear on medical students and doctors in their pre-independent professional training to

* This was made possible by a travelling fellowship from the Medicine Gilliland Foundation (administered by the Royal College of Physicians) and study leave granted by Imperial College.

accept the moral norms of the profession, of the specialty and of the particular teacher. The basic methods of this sort of medical ethics education amount essentially (to be candid if somewhat brutal) to stick–carrot or other Pavlovian techniques which ensure that the student or doctor in training is rewarded if he conforms and punished if he fails to conform to the established norms.[1] Dunstan has defined medical ethics as 'the obligations of a moral nature which govern the practice of medicine'[2] and it is this sense of medical ethics which has been traditionally taught – or 'imparted' – during medical *training* using the methods just outlined. Furthermore, it is this sense of medical ethics which is outlined in the various medical codes and declarations[3] and which is enforced by the General Medical Council[4] and other national regulatory bodies. Let us call this concept of medical ethics traditional medical ethics; it might also be called, not too misleadingly, normative medical ethics or medical morals.

The second concept of medical ethics, critical or philosophical medical ethics, is a much newer arrival in medical education. In brief, it is the *critical study* of moral problems arising in the context of medical practice. It requires analysis of the moral reasoning which underpins *any* substantive medico-moral claim, and involves consideration of counter-claims and counter-arguments. Central to philosophical medical ethics is critical study of the content of traditional medical ethics. While there can be little doubt that the medical profession has and must have particular moral obligations, including an obligation to educate its members to accept these obligations and to ensure that they behave accordingly, it seems clear that such education is inadequate if it fails to include critical scrutiny of these obligations.[5] It is now increasingly recognised that traditional medical ethics education needs to be supplemented by philosophical or critical medical ethics education. With a few exceptions, British medical schools have until very recently offered very little of the latter. In America, on the other hand, it has been rapidly introduced over the last ten to twenty years so that now formal courses in medical ethics, including at least a component of critical medical ethics, are the norm.[6]

## The American system of medical education

American medical education is divided into premedical (all American medical students have to have a university degree prior to acceptance; usually these degrees are made up of credits in a variety of subjects taken to varying levels of scholarship, depending on the student's interests and the resources of his university or college); preclinical (the first two years of medical education); and clinical (the final two years of medical education). They then take the medical final examinations and are awarded MDs if they pass (I believe that only Yale requires a doctoral dissertation as well as the final examinations). They then spend a compulsory year of internship and either immediately go into private general practice (now rather rare) or undertake some sort of specialty training, including appropriate rotation of junior posts and specialty board examinations. After they have passed the specialty board examinations they are accredited specialists and are entitled to practise independently as such.

The next four sections of this paper will consider American medical ethics teaching provision in each of the above categories: premedical, preclinical, clinical and postgraduate.

## Premedical medical ethics education

My impression – though it is no more than that – is that most universities with philosophy departments and many with theology departments are now offering courses in medical ethics at the undergraduate level in addition to their general ethics courses,[7] and that both types of course are available to all undergraduates including those who wish to apply for medical school. However, the medical schools do not generally require or give preferential consideration to applicants who have credits in ethics. Instead they put a high premium on relevant science subjects and few medical students have had much premedical teaching in ethics or humanities. Only four per cent of medical student applicants in one survey[8] had majored in humanities (and eight per cent had majored in social sciences).

## Preclinical medical ethics teaching

Provision varies widely from none at all to compulsory courses of 10-15 hours 'contact time' in each of the two preclinical years, with additional private study required, and examinations or other formal assessments. An important division exists between the small minority of medical schools teaching a variety of medical humanities subjects and those whose only – or at any rate whose predominant – humanities teaching is in medical ethics. Of the former, the longest established and most respected combined humanities programme is at Hershey in the University of Pennsylvania Medical School. It includes philosophy, theology, history, literature and the visual arts, all in relation to medicine. Another important humanities-teaching medical school is that of Georgetown University in Washington which has the assistance of the renowned Kennedy Institute of Ethics. It begins its health and humanities programme in the first preclinical year. As well as ethics (its main feature) it also includes law and medicine, literature and medicine, the history of medicine, and fine arts and medicine. A third important medical humanities programme is at the University of Texas medical branch at Galveston; its large staff has expertise in philosophy, theology, history, literature, American studies, psychology and law. Most medical schools, however, do not have such broad-ranging humanities programmes.

The content of the introductory courses in medical ethics given to preclinical students varies. Some courses start straight away with clinical cases embodying medico-moral dilemmas; sometimes the students are asked to contribute cases they have come across; more often the lecturer describes a problem case and invites discussion. Once the discussion has progressed enough for a variety of views and justifications of those views to be expressed, the lecturer may pick out some of the underlying types of moral reasoning, moral assumptions, and moral concepts and discuss them at length. Alternatively, the lecturer may start analysing a problematic case, briefly indicating the implications of the various positions outlined. Another approach is to give a few introductory lectures about different sorts of ethical theory and indicate how these may be used to try to resolve some specific medico-moral problems.

Yet another approach is to start with the Hippocratic Oath and other medical codes of ethics (such as those of the World Medical Association Declarations, the American Medical Association, and of the various specialty organisations) and then try to resolve medico-moral problems on the basis of these codes, progressing from there to some basic discussion of relevant ethical theory. It seems to be almost universally agreed that however the course starts, discussion of specific problem cases in medical ethics is essential and should be brought in early. Let me give two examples.

At the Michigan State University medical school the first-year course in medical ethics is compulsory and involves weekly three-hour sessions over a ten-week term. The first hour involves a lecture based on a case (for example, a case of a brain-dead child; the Karen Quinlan case; different sorts of requests to be allowed to die; a young woman with acute leukaemia facing a choice between hospice care and an experimental drug protocol). After the presentation the students discuss the issues in small groups each led by a physician and a non-medical member of the medical humanities programme. The emphasis is on eliciting their *reasoning* and their consideration of the implications of their position. They are taught to analyse cases by outlining the medical features, the different ethical issues involved, the alternative courses of action available and the advantages and disadvantages of each; they are required to specify further information required and why they believe it will be ethically relevant and how they would set about obtaining it. They are then asked to attempt to resolve the moral dilemma, giving their reasoning and the ethical principles or values relied on. Finally, they are asked to outline weaknesses in the position they support, and to offer at least one relevant reference to the literature. For their assessment they have to give a case presentation indicating the problem areas. This, according to Dr Howard Brody, who is both a practising and teaching family physician and a teaching professional philosopher, provides an adequate assessment of basic competence in the subject (or its absence).

## An 'ethical workup'

At the Stritch School of Medicine, Loyola University of Chicago, the first preclinical year ethics course is again compulsory and involves some thirteen contact hours. It is oriented to teaching students to make a standardised assessment of a medico-moral problem – what is known there as an 'ethical workup'. This method requires the student to describe all the facts in the case, including medical facts possibly relevant to its outcome; to describe 'relevant values' – values, that is, of the physicians, patients, housestaff, the hospital itself, and society (this is not an exhaustive list); to determine the main value clash (for example, between the doctor's desire to heal and the patient's desire for a different course of action); to determine possible courses of action which could protect as many of the values in the case as possible; to choose a course of action; and to defend the chosen course of action and the priority in this case of the values it expresses.[9] In this context it may be appropriate to mention the ethical presentation recommended to *clinical* students by the three authors of *Clinical Ethics*, all of whom teach medical ethics and encourage their method of presentation at their medical schools – at the time those of the University of California in Los Angeles and San Francisco, and at the University of Chicago.[10] Their suggested framework for presentation is: give the indications for medical intervention; discuss the patient's preferences in the case; discuss relevant 'quality of life' considerations; and discuss relevant 'external' factors (such as family considerations, costs, research values, teaching values, and the safety and wellbeing of society).

## Clinical medical ethics teaching

Most of the clinical ethics teaching I encountered was optional (elective) and was provided on particular firms or clerkships. Among the diverse offerings were: wardround discussions of ethical issues, often co-taught by the clinical teacher and a visiting philosopher/theologian/lawyer or other medical ethicist; lunchtime meetings; case conferences; seminars; so called ethics grand rounds which take the following form. A patient whose case is medico-morally complex is described briefly, usually by the resident, but sometimes by a clinical student; a clinical teacher analyses the issues as he or she sees them; and then one or more specialists in medical ethics gives a more

extended analysis of the ethical issues. Sometimes, and I
believe increasingly commonly, these analyses are followed by
the ethicist's statement of how he or she would deal or have
dealt with the case; finally there is general audience partici-
pation in the discussion.

## A two-week course

A few medical schools offer intensive short medical ethics
courses for clinical students. At the University of California at
San Francisco (where the medical ethics teaching was instituted
as a direct result of student demands – a phenomenon which I
encountered in several medical schools and which I have since
subversively encouraged interested medical students to emu-
late in Britain) a two-week course called 'Responsibilities of
Medical Practice' is mostly devoted to medical ethics, and is
compulsory for final year medical students (the course in 1984
was at the end of the medical course). It includes presentations
of medico-morally complex case-histories with discussions by
clinicians, lawyers and ethicists. The discussions include panel
discussions with audience participation and small group discussions. There is a lecture on medico-moral decision-making
(incorporating and expanding the approach outlined above and
in *Clinical Ethics*). The general categories for the rest of the
course (usually a whole day per category) are: responsibility
for care of the critically and terminally ill; responsibility to
inform; responsibility for working with colleagues; responsibility to self and family; responsibility for the health of the
nation; responsibility for the cost of medical care; responsibility for patients with complex problems; and responsibility
for the care of children. The two-week course is examined by
giving the students a medico-moral case history and asking
them to write a brief analysis as though they were writing a
progress note, outlining the important ethical features of
the case and ways of responding to these, with justifications
for their preferred approach. All participants on the course
are given a collection of 'resource material' to back up
the individual sessions, with photocopies of appropriate
journal articles and other literature (including newspaper
articles).

*Clinical ethics at the University of Chicago*

Another notable approach to clinical ethics is that at the University of Chicago Pritzker Medical School, where the medical ethics teaching was and still is largely coordinated by Dr Mark Siegler, an internist, associate professor of medicine, and a major medical contributor to the American medical ethics literature. Although Dr Siegler has involved himself in considerable postgraduate philosophical training and scholarship and appreciates the 'important contribution' that philosophers and theologians and other 'theoreticians' make to the study of medical ethics, he believes that these non-clinicians have come to dominate American medical ethics teaching excessively. At the centre of medical ethics is the clinical encounter and this, he believes, should be at the centre of medical ethics teaching. His plan, gradually coming to fruition, is to encourage a considerable number of key clinical teachers to be interested enough in medical ethics education to take some special preparation and education in the area themselves. They then develop their own teaching in medical ethics, both generally and in relation to their special areas of interest, but with the clinical encounter always its focal point. He describes his own course in the CIOMS book on medical ethics and medical education[11] but briefly, a twelve-week (originally one-month) ethics course is provided for the medical students on the medical rotation. They meet twice a week for an hour and a half (in the one-month course, three times a week) with the attending physician, a resident, and members of the other health-related disciplines – nurses, social workers, chaplains, lawyers, and occasionally theologians or philosophers.

A student – 'adhering to the highest standards of medical case presentation' – presents a case which he has found morally perplexing (or at least morally interesting). The rest of the class is encouraged to discuss the case critically. The physician generalises from the particular case, indicating the conceptual, philosophical and policy issues raised. The students are encouraged to discuss their own attitudes and their implications, including emotional or other 'affective implications'. After full discussion (at least according to the published account, although this was not mentioned to me when I visited the medical school), the presenting student is asked to give the medical firm looking after the patient a summary of the class's discussions and report back their reactions. 'We are often surprised at how a medical service will welcome and sometimes act upon suggestions which have emerged from our classroom discussions.'[11] Dr Siegler tries to ensure that cases relating to confidentiality and truth telling, to clinical decision-making in the context of doctor–patient disagreement, to decisions to prolong or not to prolong life, and to decisions concerning allocation of scarce clinical resources, are all covered in the course of the discussions.

These examples are of course from only a tiny sample of medical ethics teaching in the USA, but I have tried to select them so as to reflect some typical approaches. A more intensive analysis of eight programmes is provided by Jameton and Jonsen,[12] and a broad ranging survey of American ethics and humanities teaching in medical schools in the 1970s obtained by questionnaires and site visits is given in *Teaching Ethics, the Humanities, and Human Values in Medical Schools.*[6] An excellent discussion of medical ethics teaching is given by Clouser,[13] including a description of a typical medical ethics class. Other useful reports are listed in the notes and references at the end of this chapter.[14,15]

## Postgraduate medical ethics teaching

There seem to be three main categories of medical ethics teaching orientated towards doctors: teaching that is aimed at doctors who themselves will be teaching medical ethics to medical students and doctors in training; teaching that is aimed at doctors in training; and teaching that is aimed at the medical profession in general.

It is self-evident that medical ethics teaching in medical schools can only occur if at least some teaching doctors believe that it should be taught. I have little doubt that in America still, though less than in Britain, there is widespread agnosticism, indifference and not a little downright hostility within the medical teaching community to what I have called critical/philosophical medical ethics. It is my impression that much of this stems from misunderstanding of what critical medical ethics teaching involves. In particular there is a widespread misconception that critical medical ethics sets out to *inculcate* certain moral attitudes and moral norms. This view is false. But it is hardly surprising that doctors whose own experience has been with traditional medical ethics teaching, both as students and as teachers, should have this misconception, for traditional medical ethics *does* set out to inculcate certain attitudes and moral norms (and in my opinion entirely properly does so). Once medical teachers see that one of the main functions of critical medical ethics teaching is to *strengthen* traditional medical ethics teaching by providing a rational framework for its assessment and development many seem to be reassured – though there are, of course, those who are not prepared to submit their medico-moral positions to intellectual scrutiny or to try to justify them in the light of counter-arguments. Considerable attention has been paid to the question of how to get sufficient teaching doctors interested enough in critical/ philosophical medical ethics to begin to find out what it really involves. A wide range of methods has been deployed.

## *Learning by teaching*

Perhaps the most common approach is the familiar medical strategy of learning by teaching. Thus wily enthusiasts seek the aid of *interested* medical colleagues to co-teach. Normally in America (though of course it may be the other way around) this seems to involve a non-medical ethicist asking a doctor whom he knows to be interested in medical ethics to allow him to sit in on a class in which medical ethics is likely to arise. The response probably depends on the relationship between the two. If the doctor knows, likes and trusts the ethicist personally he will accept with alacrity; if not, there may be considerable wariness (largely based, I suspect, on the misconception noted above, but also on a considerable fear that the ethicist is going to make the doctor look foolish or tie him up in intellectual knots). Once the ethicist has his foot in the door there is usually a more or less gradual development into co-teaching, and both partners find they learn a lot from each other. Not infrequently they will meet to discuss a class beforehand and iron out potential problems, especially of medical pitfalls facing the philosopher or theologian and philosophical problems facing the doctor. The usual pattern of such co-teaching seems to be case-based, with the co-teachers encouraging the students (whoever they are) to analyse the cases along the same sorts of lines as those outlined above for teaching clinical students. The co-teachers then clarify and distinguish the arguments being used, discuss the concepts involved, add additional arguments for and against positions, generalise the themes being expressed, elicit the principles or values being relied on, develop the implications of different positions for other cases, often apparently unrelated, and then return to the specific case in an attempt to achieve what the Americans call 'closure' (a decision about what should be done). This sort of approach can be adapted to a wide variety of contexts, and in practice seems to be used on routine clinical ward rounds (at different levels); on grand rounds given over specifically to medico-moral analysis (the ethics grand rounds described above); at lectures and seminars; and at lunchtime meetings ('brownbaggers').

Another way of involving teaching doctors is to lay on large meetings for the hospital population (with or without partici-pation from the surrounding community) in which specific issues in medical ethics are debated: the enthusiast then asks some interested clinical teachers to come along and contribute their own analyses and the prospect of so doing often encourages some homework beforehand. Such meetings may be very similar to those at The London Hospital and other medical groups in Britain and their popularity varies.

*Ethics consultation services*

Another way of involving clinicians in critical medical ethics is by providing an ethics consultation service; doctors faced with a medico-morally complex problem can ask to consult the ethicist. Some hospitals have hired philosophers to provide them with consultation facilities and to provide general medical ethics education using the same sorts of techniques as described above. Interestingly, the consultation service is often seen as a two-edged sword by the ethicists I spoke to. If it is used by the doctors as a means of clarifying the arguments, the dilemmas, the concepts, the implications of different positions, then they believe they are providing a useful and appropriate service. Some doctors, however, tended to try to use the ethics consultation service as a way of saving time, avoiding difficult decisions, or 'generally passing the moral buck'. That is precisely what such ethicists are anxious to avoid; they see themselves as helping doctors to make their own medico-moral decisions more rigorously; they positively reject (and I believe that this rejection is genuine) any invitation to take over the decision-making. This provides an important response to worries often voiced by British doctors that ethics consultation services would undermine clinical responsibility. Provided that philosophers/ethicists are chosen who are not by person-ality inclined to 'take over', the main problem seems less likely to be one of philosophers undermining clinical responsibility so much as preventing some doctors from trying to hand over ethical decision-making, much as they typically do when they ask other specialists for their opinions. For while it may be appropriate simply to do what the dermatologist recom-mends in the bottom line of his consulting note, it is inappropriate (I here simply assert) to try to use an ethics consultation in the same way. Thus part of the function of ethics consultants may well have to be to remind those doctors who wish to hand over ethical decision-making about the moral problems of doing so!

Some medical schools offer rather more thorough academic analysis of medical ethics, and the intensity of this varies across the spectrum from the occasional lecture to a PhD course.

*Short intensive courses*

Various short intensive courses in medical ethics are available to interested doctors. Perhaps the best known of these (though it has now been discontinued because funds from the National Endowment for the Humanities have dried up) was the four-to six-week full-time summer course offered in Washington and elsewhere by, among others, William May, Tristram Engelhardt, Leon Kass, James Childress and Sam Gorovitz. Many of the doctors currently involved in medical ethics teaching have been on one of these very intensive courses on philosophical medical ethics or other humanities and I have heard nothing but the highest praise for them.

Less ambitions, one-week courses are run every summer by the Kennedy Institute and in some years by the Hastings Center. They provide a shortened but equally intensive introduction to critical/philosophical medical ethics (and, indeed, our own annual intensive course in medical ethics for nursing and medical teachers held at Imperial College each September is significantly modelled on the Kennedy Institute course). More prolonged training in medical ethics is provided by a variety of formal academic courses; interdisciplinary university seminars; MA degrees in medical ethics, such as that offered at Stritch School of Medicine in Chicago (and the one-year MA in medical ethics which, I understand, is being developed at Harvard); and, for the real enthusiasts, PhDs. Other facilities include one- or two-year fellowships such as those offered at UCSF and at the University of Texas at Galveston in which doctors can develop their understanding of the philosophical and/or theological aspects of medical ethics.

Similar courses are now being developed in Britain: the Apothecaries diploma course in the philosophy of medicine (which started in 1978) being followed by a diploma and then MA in medical law and ethics at Kings College London; a highly popular MA in health care ethics at the University of Wales which can be done by people all over the country while they continue their work; an MA in health care ethics at the University of Manchester; an MSc in medical ethics in the University of Liverpool; and a diploma in medical ethics at the University of Keele. Doubtless others will have been created by the time this is read.

It seems widely agreed among medical ethics doctors and 'humanists' (in American English this means academics whose university education has been in the humanities) that some sort of additional training for a small proportion of medical teachers who are particularly interested in teaching medical ethics is desirable.

A tendency is just discernible for critical medical ethics education to be provided to doctors training for specialty board examinations, and I understand that the internal medicine board now includes (critical) medical ethics questions in its syllabus, and that the paediatrics, family medicine and obstetrics/gynaecology boards are considering doing so. One course for residents, organised by Dr Tom Elkins at the University of Tennessee Medical Center, in association with the medical ethicists there, required obstetrics/gynaecology housestaff in their first year to attend three one-hour sessions a week for three weeks, all devoted to medical ethics, and involving a mixture of traditional and critical medical ethics. Despite the fact that the sessions began at seven in the morning, Dr Elkins assured me that it was very popular among the housestaff. At the University of Chicago Medical Center a recently qualified medical graduate made what seemed to me to be an important point: if medical students were taught (critical) medical ethics while their housemen and residents were not, there was a considerable likelihood of the medical ethics teaching being rapidly undermined by the cynicism and otherwise negative responses of their immediate bosses. 'If physicians don't know about something they tend to discount it.'

So far as medical ethics education for the medical profession at large is concerned, relatively little seemed to be provided over and above the sorts of programmes sketched above. However, continuing education programmes at some centres include sessions devoted to medical ethics – though my impression is that these sessions tend to be more in the traditional medical ethics category than critical/philosophical. Judging by one such postgraduate refresher course I attended there would be little enthusiasm from participants for the latter.

The various tactics used to evoke doctors' interest in medical ethics included the following approximate quotations from medical ethics professionals, medical and non-medical, whom I interviewed. 'Get them talking about cases and show them how full of ethical issues most of them are.' 'Point out to them that they don't have to reinvent the wheel. A lot of these issues have been very thoroughly thought through already.' 'Warn them that if they don't get serious about medical ethics, society will do it for them.' 'Remind them that doctors are actually contributing to a sicker society by keeping ill people alive who would otherwise have died, and at the same time imposing an enormous financial burden on society. So it's their responsibility to think very critically about the ethics of what they are doing.' 'Remind them repeatedly that you aren't there to moralise or criticise but to analyse.' Tell them about the legal situation and slip in a bit of ethical analysis while you're there' (this from a lawyer-ethicist). 'Above all keep it clinical. Of course some theory is needed, but it has to explain the clinical situation.'

'Avoid abstractions and weird philosophers' examples – doctors are very concrete thinkers.' 'Don't play intellectual games with doctors or make them feel foolish. It might work with philosophy undergraduates, but not with medical students let alone doctors.' 'Never call what you're doing physician education. Of course it is, but call it faculty enhancement.' 'Make it clear that you respect, indeed admire doctors, and what they are doing.' 'Doctor haters need not apply.' 'If you want to reform the system don't go in for medical ethics.'

## Objectives of medical ethics education

A point worth reiterating, time and time again I suspect, is that I did not meet a single medical ethics teacher in America who wanted either to take over ethical decision-making from doctors or to indoctrinate or otherwise coerce doctors into making the sort of moral decisions of which they, the educators, personally approved. Rather, the medical ethicists were unanimous in seeing themselves as offering skills of various sorts which would enable doctors to improve *their own* medico-moral decision-making. This is not to deny, of course, that the medical ethics teachers *had* their own views about what sorts of medico-moral decisions doctors ought to be making; it is to deny that they wanted to impose those views on the medical students and doctors they taught.

### Critical medico-moral thinking and discursive moral competence

One skill which all the medical ethicists I met unanimously agreed to be necessary was *clear thinking about medico-moral issues*. From time to time, the contrast was pointed out between the rigour required in technical and scientific aspects of medical education and the sloppiness and woolliness of thought apparently acceptable in traditional medical ethics education. The sorts of clear thinking promoted by medical ethics teachers include logical, unambiguous argument (and correspondingly the detection of ambiguous, fallacious or otherwise confused argument); conceptual clarity; the identification and understanding of moral principles or values being used in an argument or chain of reasoning, and the ability to distinguish these from (merely) technical, scientific, instrumental and other, non-moral, considerations; consistency; and the ability to discern the implications of moral claims and arguments for different contexts. These components should not seem mysterious for they are those of *any* basic education in moral reasoning – though of course, particular attention is paid to them in philosophy, law and theology. They can be summarised by the term 'critical moral thinking'. Most American medical ethics teachers teach this in the context of medico-moral issues, recognising that the primary objective of such critical moral thinking in the context of *medical* education is to help doctors think critically about the moral aspects of *medical* practice. I think it would be fair to say that critical thinking about the moral aspects of medical practice constitutes the bulk of what William Ruddick, Professor of Philosophy at New York University, sees as the primary objective of medical ethics education – what he calls 'discursive moral competence' (the ability to identify and discuss moral matters with a variety of colleagues, patients, their families, and others). Incidentally, perhaps I should add another component of this discursive moral competence which several medical ethicists emphasised: opposition to over-simplification. Ruth Macklin, Professor of Medical Ethics at Albert Einstein College of Medicine in New York, spoke for all when she quoted some sage or other: 'Everything should be simplified as far as possible – and no further'.

## Medical humanities and medical ethics teaching

While all medical ethicists would I think agree that critical medico-moral thinking is a *necessary* part of medical ethics education, there is disagreement about whether it is *sufficient*. Proponents of the medical humanities approach would add, as a second objective in medical ethics education, a variety of other skills aimed to make the doctor-to-be more imaginative (particularly more morally imaginative), more empathetic with a wide variety of people (particularly with a wide variety of suffering people), and more ready and able to tolerate ambiguity, disagreement and moral conflict. The DeCamp conference on basic curricular goals in medical ethics specified various 'interactional skills' that its members, all active in teaching biomedical ethics, believed were essential. These included being able to talk sensitively with patients about terminal illness, about resuscitation plans, or about other potentially distressing matters, and being able to convey clearly and 'in language which a patient can understand' appropriate information necessary to obtain informed consent.[16]

It seems to me that, as far as medical ethics teaching is concerned, the common objective of this seemingly disparate group of disciplines and skills, called in America 'medical humanities', can be summarised as a desire to enhance the doctor's understanding of, and ability to respond to, non-cognitive aspects of his patients' and his own moral beliefs, attitudes and behaviour, including the social, cultural and psychological factors which may influence them.

## Normative medical ethics teaching

A third group of objectives to be discerned in American medical ethics education have the common feature of being normative – that is to say of establishing and promoting moral norms or standards. While, as I have stated, none of the medical ethics teachers I interviewed wished to take over medico-moral decision-making from doctors, or indoctrinate or otherwise coerce students or doctors into decisions of which they would personally approve, there is no doubt in my mind that a substantial proportion do wish to help establish and promote certain moral norms and standards and to disestablish and discourage others. Daniel Callahan, Director of the Hastings Center and a philosopher with a theological background, hopes his reading in other subjects has saved him 'from some of the worst traits of pure philosophers'. He is explicit that philosophical rigour is necessary but not sufficient for an adequate medical ethics education, and that some basic moral norms – including a sense of obligation not only to patients but also to society, as well as respect for people's autonomy – should be actively encouraged in medical ethics programmes. And he adds the important (to non-medical teachers) reminder that the purpose of medical ethics education in medical schools is not to train up good moral philosophers but to improve the education of good *doctors*. In this regard he told me he believed that 'the teacher of medical

ethics has himself to strive to be, as far as possible, something
of an ethical role model – at least in trying to convey what it
means to be a sensitive, thoughtful and observant human
being. He should try in his own conduct to convey to others
the kind of respect that patients are due.'

I don't think that many of the ethicists I met would dissent
from all that, although they would, I believe, vary somewhat
about how 'active' they should be in encouraging these norms.
On the whole I think that at least those with philosophical
backgrounds, and probably most of the others too, would tend
to confine their 'activity' to the use of reasoned argument; they
would agree with Jameton and Jonsen that 'philosophers are so
unwilling to indoctrinate, and indoctrination is so antithetical
to most notions of education, that it should be ruled out as a
goal' and 'the moral "policing" of medicine is too much to ask
of ethics teaching'.[17] They would also agree with the participants in the DeCamp conference who believe that 'a medical
ethics curriculum is designed not to improve the moral
character of future physicians, but to provide those of sound
moral character with the intellectual tools and interactional
skills with which to determine its best behavioural expression'.[16]
However, I suspect that a few individuals exist in medical
ethics teaching who are not averse to moral arm-twisting,
indoctrination and 'moral policing'. I believe that we would do
well to look out for such characters and avoid appointing them
to medical ethics teaching posts as (and if) these become
established in Britain.

There is a substantial problem here. Such characters share an
approach and attitude not uncommon among medical teachers
who often use such methods in their ordinary medical teaching
and who, at least if reason alone is not effective in producing
the desired moral outlook and/or behaviour, feel not just
permitted but obliged to coerce their students into conformity
with the threat of ultimate expulsion. An obvious example
would be as follows. It is not part of a philosophy teacher's
business to prevent his students from going to bed with other
people. However, it *is* part of a medical teacher's business to
prevent his students sleeping with patients; and while (so I
would argue) sound moral reasoning to explain this prohibition, with appropriate subjection of such reasoning to counter-
arguments, should be an important component of medical

ethics education, so too is the normative socialisation of medical students and doctors characteristic of traditional medical ethics. The determination of the moral norms of the profession should be subject to critical moral thinking, but the moral norms need to be instilled and, if necessary, enforced. How should we resolve the dilemma?

It is in this context that the distinction between the two concepts of medical ethics is most important (traditional or normative medical ethics and critical or philosophical medical ethics) for their objectives are different. My own view is that traditional medical ethics – the inculcation, indoctrination and enforcement of medical ethics ('the obligations of a moral nature which govern the practice of medicine') – should be kept separate from the teaching of philosophical medical ethics, and that it should continue to be carried out by doctors in the traditional ways. I think it would be idle to pretend that such inculcation does not already exist in medical education, and I would argue (though here do not do so) that it is right that it should exist. It should however be subject, so I believe, to constant critical evaluation. Better education in critical/philosophical medical ethics should help to ensure that only those obligations (and also only those ways of inculcating and enforcing them) which have and can be shown to have strong moral justifications, and which stand up to counter-argument, are accepted by the profession as a whole.

## Unfinished agenda

I shall finish by listing, with very brief comments, the headings under which further reporting and analysis seem worthwhile.

### Assessment and evaluation of medical ethics teaching

Two distinct questions arise here: what changes are in fact produced by medical ethics teaching and do these changes make for better doctors? There is some work going on in the United States to try to answer the first question. The second question is widely considered untestable (though most enthusiasts – and I am one of them – think the answer is 'yes'. People have not, as far as I am aware, tested to find out if knowing some basic biochemistry makes people better doctors. They assume that doctors who understand the rationale underlying their actions are better doctors than those who do not. In both cases the assumptions *may* be false but it seems reasonable to accept them as true.) Ideally it would be helpful to know what the students, the doctors and the patients think about this second question, but we are unlikely ever to find out. As far as the first is concerned, the study by Pellegrino and associates[18] obtained questionnaire responses from about 1000 recent medical graduates about their perceptions of medical ethics teaching. Although most of the 300 or so respondents who had had formal medical ethics teaching perceived a variety of inadequacies, about 70–80 per cent (depending on the specific questions) found it to be 'very or somewhat successful' in helping them identify value conflicts, increase their sensitivity to patients' needs, understand their own values better, and deal more openly with moral dilemmas, both with their patients and with their fellow professionals.

Among the studies I came across was the report by Jameton and Jonsen[12] and the medical ethics teaching evaluation project at the Michigan State University medical, osteopathic nursing and veterinary schools.[19]

## Who should teach medical ethics?

There is considerable discussion about this. At present it is taught by academics with a wide variety of backgrounds, but predominantly by doctors, philosophers and theologians, with lawyers, sociologists, psychologists, historians and teachers of literature comprising a small minority. In the Society for Health and Human Values survey of 114 medical schools,[6] nearly half the 1064 teachers of medical ethics were reported to be doctors. However, doctors also made up the bulk of the 57 per cent of medical ethics teachers who spent less than 10 per cent of their time in teaching medical ethics.

There does seem to be agreement that the best way of teaching the subject is by co-teaching – that is, with a medical teacher and ethicist sharing the teaching, preferably together. However, this is recognised to be a very *expensive* way of teaching. I am personally attracted to Dr Siegler's approach at the University of Chicago Medical School (shared in one form or another by many of the ethicists I met, medical and non-medical) whereby a core of medical teachers acquire expertise in ethics by means of courses, personal contacts, study, and co-teaching, and then take on the bulk of clinical ethics teaching. In addition I would agree with a view expressed by two different doctors *not* involved in medical ethics teaching that there should be a small cadre of doctors trained more thoroughly in ethics and medical ethics who should teach within the medical schools but also do research within the disciplines of moral philosophy, moral theology, law and medical ethics, and so on. These doctors would function as links between the parent academic disciplines and medical teachers, practitioners and students, rather like the doctor scientists who perform a similar function for the various medical sciences.

There is general agreement among all the people to whom I spoke about medical ethics teaching in the USA (although it was a biased sample) that medical ethics teaching has to be, in some way, a multidisciplinary activity. But a variety of ways of incorporating non-doctors has been advocated and these deserve more consideration than I have offered.

## A military approach to ethics teaching

Perhaps I should mention briefly the approach of another profession, the military, which, like the medical profession (at least in its hospital sector), is intensely hierarchical. I had heard at a philosophy conference in England that the American military had begun to teach military ethics and so I followed this up by visiting West Point Military Academy and interviewing Colonel Anthony Hartle who is in charge of its philosophy and military ethics teaching. He thinks he is the only philosophy PhD in the American Army and he obtained the degree at the instigation of the Army authorities who had decided to institute professional teaching of military ethics. He was then appointed to the West Point Military Academy permanent staff to set up a programme. He now has 12 officers helping him with this teaching, each of whom is on a five-year 'tour'. They each spend two years in a university acquiring an MA in philosophy with an emphasis on ethics and then three years teaching military ethics on Colonel Hartle's programme before passing on to some other military tour of duty. The

Academy has a core programme in ethics which each cadet must pass. It assists the cadets with the syllabus of their own classes in the 'honour code' and runs a variety of elective programmes in philosophy and ethics. In addition, the Academy is in the process of building up a core programme of ethics teaching for various courses which officers are required to take as they climb the military hierarchy. The efficiency of the staff preparation for ethics classes at West Point must be unrivalled. Each teaching officer has a book outlining the syllabus *for each class* which details all the equipment needed – not merely the audiovisual equipment, but dusters and chalk too! The possibility of emulating the US Army not only in such efficiency but also in offering five-year specialty tours of medical ethics teaching duty – two years for training and three years for teaching – may be worth considering for British medical ethics teaching.

*Training of medical ethics teachers*

I have discussed at some length the training in the USA of doctors interested in teaching medical ethics and indicated that it was generally agreed that they needed *some* special education in ethics. 'Enthusiasm, good will and interest are not sufficient qualifications for teaching courses in organic chemistry, microeconomics or Greek literature. There is no reason why they should be thought sufficient for the teaching of ethics, a difficult subject with a long history.'[20] Conversely, it is widely recognised that experience of clinical medicine is essential for anyone purporting to teach medical ethics, and the Hastings Center report on the teaching of ethics in higher education also recommends at least a year of some sort of medical education for non-doctors, taken *en bloc* or accumulatively.[20] Several courses leading to PhDs in medical ethics which include clinical experience now exist in America. There are also some MAs and Harvard University is, I understand, planning a one-year course for graduates from different disciplines who are interested in teaching medical ethics, tailoring individual programmes designed to help fill the relevant gaps in their previous education. In this respect I think we in Britain should seriously consider developing Sir Douglas Black's idea and open up our medical schools to philosophers, theologians, lawyers and others interested in studying medical ethics, with a view to giving them an introductory course, similar to that given to clinical students, and an opportunity to experience any aspects of clinical medicine which interest them.[21]

## Methods of teaching medical ethics

A further aspect of training for medical ethics teachers is methodology: which methods of teaching are most successful? Considerable variation is to be found in America, and it is an area which we in Britain would be wise to look into, preferably *before* setting up programmes, as bad teaching can obviously contribute to the failure of any such programmes. I have listed various bits of advice given to me to make such teaching more attractive to doctors at the end of the section on postgraduate medical ethics teaching. In addition, the following features should be vigorously avoided: long lectures; lack of clinical material; lack of opportunity for discussion; excessive and inaccessible reference material; excessive theory divorced from clinical examples; courses given by a variety of one-off lecturers, especially if the lectures have not been previously coordinated by the course organiser; allowing excessive clinical anecdotes to swamp discussion; excessive concern with legal aspects of ethical issues; inadequate understanding that *acrimony* is not an acceptable aspect of medical ethics, however strong the disagreement.

A useful discussion of medical ethics teaching methods is given by Clouser.[22]

## Setting up medical ethics teaching programmes – practicalities

The following are a few hints I was offered (approximate verbatim quotes). 'Have a long development and preparation for any programme. Consult widely, preferably with a variety of clinical teachers, with medical students, with different sectors of health care provision and preferably too with representatives of the local community.' 'Hire teachers on at least a year's probation and let them go [American for 'sack them'] if they are not successful'. 'Consult with people who have done it; you'll save yourself a lot of effort.' 'The advice of the Society for Health and Human Values team was invaluable' (perhaps the British centres already involved in teaching medical ethics in Britain should consider offering others the help of advisory teams?). 'Hire teachers who *like* doctors and medicine.' 'Avoid young and inexperienced teachers for setting up programmes; you'll need all the skill and experience you can find.' 'Get a politically strong clinical department to introduce and positively support a new medical ethics programme.' 'Avoid spreading your teaching too thin; it will get a bad name.' 'Get the philosophers to quote from the great philosophers; philosophers too often sound like intelligent laymen, and that doesn't impress doctors' (sic). 'You'll probably have to start with voluntary teaching; if so make it clear that the unpaid teaching will last so long and no longer.' 'Make sure that your teachers do not take on too great a load; they must have time for reflection, research and contact with their base discipline.' 'Don't worry if you can't start with a perfect programme; settle for a good one even if it is not as good as you'd want.'

A moderately useful discussion concerning the setting up of programmes, called 'Priorities for Teaching Bioethics' is given in the Hastings Center's *The Teaching of Bioethics*.[14]

My own medical ethics teaching has certainly profited from some of the advice I was given in America – both about what to do and what to avoid. I can only hope that this rather extensive but incomplete account of what I learnt about American medical ethics teaching, will also be of some help to those in Britain and other countries now beginning to set up teaching programmes in philosophical medical ethics.[23]

## Notes and references

1 A fascinating account of such processes is given by a sociologist who spent 18 months living with and observing a group of American trainee surgeons. See C L Bosk. Forgive and remember: managing medical failure. Chicago, University of Chicago Press, 1979.

2 A S Duncan, G R Dunstan and R B Welbourn (eds). Dictionary of medical ethics (2nd edition). London, Darton, Longman and Todd, 1981, page xxviii.

3 See, for instance, entries under 'Declarations' and 'Hippocratic oath' in Dictionary of medical ethics (see 2 above).

4 General Medical Council. Professional conduct and discipline: fitness to practise. London, General Medical Council, 1987.

5 I have argued more fully for the need for education in critical or philosophical medical ethics in R Gillon. The function of criticism. British Medical Journal, 283, 1981, pages 1633–1639.

6 E D Pellegrino and T K McElhinney. Teaching ethics, the humanities, and human values in medical schools: a ten-year overview. Washington DC, Society for health and human values, 1981. Available from G K Degnon Associates Inc, McLean, Virginia 22101, USA.

7 'We estimate that at least 11,000–12,000 courses in ethics are currently taught at the undergraduate and professional school levels.' The Hastings Center. The teaching of ethics in higher education. Hastings on Hudson, The Hastings Center, 1980. (All the Center's publications are available from 255 Elm Road, Briarcliff Manor, NY 10510, USA.)

8 J T Bruer and K S Warren. Liberal arts and the premedical curriculum. Journal of the American Medical Association, 245, 1981, pages 364–366.

9 D C Thomasma, personal communication. Professor Thomasma would be happy to correspond with interested inquirers. His address is: Director, Medical Humanities Department, Loyola University, Stritch School of Medicine, 2160 South First Avenue, Maywood, Illinois 60153, USA.

10 A R Jonsen, M Siegler and W J Winslade. Clinical ethics. London, Baillière Tindall, 1982, pages 5–8.

11 M Siegler. Medical ethics instruction for medical students in the clinical years. In: Z Bankowski and J Corvera Bernardelli (eds). Medical ethics and medical education. Geneva, CIOMS, 1981, pages 196–210. (Available from HMSO.)

12 A J Jameton and A R Jonsen. The evaluation of curriculum in medical ethics in schools of medicine. Report to the National Endowment for the Humanities and the Josiah Macy Jr Foundation, 1984. (A J Jameton can be contacted at the Institute for Health Policy Studies, School of Medicine, 1326 Third Avenue, San Francisco, California 94143, USA.)

13 K D Clouser. Teaching bioethics: strategies, problems, and resources. Hastings on Hudson, The Hastings Center, 1980.

14 See The Hastings Center. The teaching of medical ethics. Hastings on Hudson, The Hastings Center, 1972. (This is a

particularly interesting multidisciplinary collection of papers given at a large conference of American medical school teachers in the early days of the development in America of medical ethics as an academic subject.) See also The teaching of bioethics: report of the Commission on the Teaching of Bioethics, 1976; The teaching of ethics in higher education, 1980; Ethics teaching in higher education, 1980. All obtainable from The Hastings Center (see 7 above for address).

15 There is considerable American literature on medical ethics education. In addition to publications specifically cited, an interesting account of philosophical and legal perspectives on teaching medical ethics in medical centres is given in W Ruddick (ed). Philosophers in medical centers. New York, Society for Philosophy and Public Affairs, 1980 (obtainable from the Society, c/o the editor, Department of Philosophy, New York University, New York, NY 10012, USA). There are also several useful short articles on American medical ethics education in W T Reich (ed). Encyclopedia of bioethics, London and New York, Collier Macmillan, 1978. And for real enthusiasts a computer search provided by the Kennedy Institute of Medical Ethics' Library – almost certainly the best medical ethics library in the world – yielded 15 non-journal references and 38 journal references. The library is at The Joseph and Rose Kennedy Institute of Ethics, Georgetown University, Washington DC 20057, USA.

16 C M Culver, K D Clouser, B Gert and others. Basic curricular goals in medical ethics (the DeCamp Conference on the Teaching of Medical Ethics). New England Journal of Medicine, 312, 4, 1985, pages 253–256.

17 See 12 above, pages 28 and 30.

18 E D Pellegrino, R J Hart, S R Henderson and others. Relevance and utility of courses in medical ethics: a survey of physician perceptions. Journal of the American Medical Association 1985 January 4. 253(1):49–53.

19 Details of the three-year investigation into evaluation of medical ethics teaching at Michigan State University are, I believe, un-published. I was given the second annual report from the evaluation team to the National Endowment for the Humanities which awarded the grant, and it contains useful details about their methods of evaluation. Correspondence could be directed to Mr Ken Howe, Medical Ethicist, Medical Humanities Program, A106 East Fee Hall, Michigan State University, East Lansing, Michigan 48824.

20 See 14 above (The teaching of ethics in higher education), pages 63 and 64.

21 Sir Douglas Black. Commentary: we need to take a fresh look at medical research. Journal of Medical Ethics, 8, 1982, page 77. See also Medicine and moral philosophy (editorial). Journal of Medical Ethics, 9, 1983, pages 3–4.

22 See 13 above, pages 19–29.

23 This chapter was extracted from the voluminous notes of my American tour so patiently typed for me by my secretary at the Journal of Medical Ethics, Mrs Maureen Bannatyne. I take this opportunity to thank her for all her work. I also thank the large number of American medical ethics teachers who gave so unstintingly of their time in educating me about what they do.

# The allocation of scarce medical resources: a democrat's dilemma

Albert Weale

Sometimes in the National Health Service (NHS) an event like the following happens. An elderly patient presents with end-stage renal failure. Dialysis is the only procedure by which this patient's life can be prolonged. The hospital renal unit is currently working at full capacity. There is no prospect of extra nurses being assigned to the work because the health authority is already at the limit of its budget and there is no source from which the increase in wages could be paid, even if the trained staff were available to manage dialysis. The patient is not well-supported domestically, and has an attitude which is unco-operative. The patient is told (falsely) that the condition cannot be treated, and a few months later dies. The unit is as well managed as any other in the service, and the other units would have made the same decision. Care has been denied because insufficient resources have been allocated to finance it.[1]

Because it involves a life or death decision, end-stage renal failure is one of the most dramatic examples of what a shortage of resources can mean. It is also a well-documented one. International comparison shows for example that the United Kingdom dialyses a smaller proportion of its over-55s than other developed countries.[2] But, though dramatic, end-stage renal failure is not unique. Treatments affecting the quality of life are also severely rationed through lack of resources. Waiting lists for elective surgery are long in the UK, and a quarter of all hip replacements are now carried out in the private sector. Such figures do not, however, give a complete picture of how deterioration in the quality of treatment, due to a persistent lack of resources, affects patients (even if it does them no detectable harm), let alone capture the effects on morale of staff and patients in shabby and out-of-date buildings.

But resources are not endless. At some point, the claims of medical advance and treatment need to be brought into balance with the resources that can be afforded. It is this issue of the balance between medical care needs and the overall volume of resources devoted to meeting those needs which this chapter will be concerned with. There are, of course, many other ethical issues that touch upon the problems of allocating scarce medical resources, including the problems of how any total that is allocated should be distributed between different uses or patient groups, or whose responsibility it is to ensure the efficient and effective use of those resources once allocated. However, it should be clear that the problem of determining the overall total of resources is one that is sufficiently complex and demanding to be treated on its own.

The opening example presented this task as the doctor's dilemma. In this paper I aim to show that it is really the democrat's dilemma, using the term democrat to refer to anyone who believes that the authority of government is ultimately based upon its discharging an obligation of accountability to the body of citizens. If the dilemma is currently experienced as a burden upon individual physicians and nursing staff, this is the result of a defect in our political and policy institutions. Or at least so I shall argue. The democrat's task is to show how the allocation of scarce medical resources between the worthy ends that compete for such resources should be conducted in a way that is morally tolerable. In proposing this argument I shall distinguish between two versions of democracy. These two versions I shall label 'responsive' government and 'responsible' government. Only responsible government, I shall argue, is able to accomplish the task of showing how an allocation of resources is justified. But before advancing this argument I need to clear up some preliminary points.

## Preliminaries

In what follows I shall be solely concerned with arguments that pertain to public medical care systems, designating by this term

those patterns of health care in which the government accepts
that its role is to ensure provision for the mass of citizens. The
governments of all developed countries, except the United
States, accept this as a responsibility of government, although
the means they use to fulfil their responsibilities vary from
direct provision via state owned and managed facilities to the
regulation of private or occupationally-based health insurance.
These differences of means, for the purposes of the present
argument, are less important than the common fact that there is
a widespread acceptance of the notion that it is the task of
government to ensure the provision of health care for the mass
of citizens and not simply the indigent poor. It is the
acceptance of this task which distinguishes modern welfare
states from their poor law predecessors.

The reasons why governments have been willing to assume
this task are various. There is certainly no one single argument
which would point to the reasons. However, a prominent
consideration is the existence of 'market failure' in the medical
care market. This exists when a market fails to exhibit the
properties that are necessary for it to achieve an optimal
allocation of goods and services – that is, one that leaves
everyone at the point where an improvement in their
economic welfare would be at the expense of someone else's.
Market failure exists to some degree in every market, and to a
significant degree in many. Its chief source in the medical care
market stems from the uncertainty that consumers experience
when they try to purchase good buys from physicians,
combined with the fact that although patients initiate health
care episodes, it is doctors who control the call upon resources.
There are purely efficiency-based arguments, therefore, for
public intervention in the medical care market, and these
supplement the common fairness arguments that point to the
unequal access to a crucial resource that would be experienced
if medicine were treated like washing powder or cornflakes.
So, for a variety of reasons, the assumption that we are dealing
with a public matter, both in fact and in principle, is well
justified.[3]

Some people say that this dilemma need not exist. No
medical care system, writes Robert Evans,[4] ought to confront
patients with the choice of your money or your life, and he
goes on to argue that modern medical care systems should be

able to deliver life-saving treatments to all who need them. In a similar vein, Fritz Beske[5] says that members of West Germany's statutory health insurance system have unlimited access to the whole range of medical and dental care. On this account, the rationing that takes place within the NHS is simply a consequence of an institutional and political fact about UK health care – namely, that it is under-resourced relative to other systems and relative to what is needed.

How far is this a plausible assumption? Suppose, for the sake of argument, that the UK's system was under-resourced. It does not follow from this claim that it is possible to institute a system of medical care that dispenses with the need to ration resources; even when access is unlimited, there is still implicit rationing within the system. Suppose it is true that no patient in Germany or Canada is ever denied access to needed treatment. It is equally true that there are some patients who do not receive needed treatment because the requisite investment has not taken place to finance the technology that would be essential to give them appropriate treatment. As long as there are still medical discoveries to be made, there is always implicit rationing of medical resources since more could be spent to improve practice beyond its current limits.

Of course it is not implied by the claim that some rationing has to take place in any medical care system that the UK's current mode and level of rationing is the right one. But that leads immediately to the third preliminary point: how might we establish what is the right mode and level? Here I shall merely have to make an assertion. Political philosophy (which is the branch of intellectual activity best equipped to cope with this question) will not yield principles that will enable us to judge whether any particular allocation of resources is the right one. It will provide a vocabulary in which we can discuss the 'basic structure' of a resource allocation process, but it will not be sufficiently detailed, or able to take into account the relevant range of circumstances, to provide principles that can be applied in any direct way to specific allocations within that structure.[6] The reason for this, in essence, is that such allocations are likely to involve detailed particular considerations which, because of their complexity, are simply ignored by general principles. In contrast, the basic structure of resource allocating institutions is something to which general principles can be applied.

The task, then, is to describe an institutional structure that would be capable of making morally defensible decisions on the allocation of scarce medical resources. To do this, I suggest, we need the distinction between responsive and responsible government.

### Responsive government *What the people want!*

The conception of democratic government as responsive rests upon the idea that the task of government is to satisfy the wants of its citizens. It can do this directly, for example, by providing goods and services, or indirectly, for example, by ensuring that markets function efficiently. Responsive government requires a mechanism for collecting information on the wants or preferences of citizens and then turning this information into a social or collective choice. One way of doing this is by the mechanism of voting. So the paradigm of political activity on this analysis is voting, and the function of a voting system is to record the wants or preferences of people and translate them into a social choice over the implementation of public policies.

We can contrast this conception of politics and democracy with the notion of responsible government. Here the basic idea is of government not as want-regarding but as reason-respecting. On this account, the task of government is not merely to respond to the wishes that are expressed but to convince the members of society that a particular course of action is the right one (or, at least, the best one all things considered). The paradigm of political activity in this conception is not voting but discussion. Politics is thought of as a process by which public discussion takes place about the issues that confront society, and the task of the government is both to make a decision about policy and to justify that decision in a forum of public debate. Voting may be necessary as a device for cutting short discussion when practical affairs press, but that is a concession to the need for action. The ideal remains discussion leading to consensus, or at least recognition by all sides that the path chosen was in some sense a justifiable one.[7]

The conception of want-regarding responsive government is deeply embedded in our current practices and thinking. Its historical antecedents can be found in the utilitarian conception of government, especially as popularised in the early nineteenth century by James Mill. More importantly, perhaps, it often remains a good description of how government is conducted. It leads to parallels between markets and politics in which both are seen as devices for satisfying wants. Schumpeter put the point with his customary trenchancy:

Politically speaking, the man is still in the nursery who has not absorbed, so as never to forget, the saying attributed to one of the most successful politicians that ever lived: 'What businessmen do not understand is that exactly as they are dealing in oil so I am dealing in votes.'[8]

Yet, despite the appeal of the notion of responsive government as a description of political processes, it remains a poor model for the manner in which governments ought to make decisions on the allocation of medical resources. To see why, consider a simplified example.

Let us suppose that a political community operates in the spirit of the responsive model of democracy. Its members vote upon the level of resources to be devoted to the supply of medical resources within the community. We imagine that they are instituting or reviewing a health care system in which they are to participate; that they are contemplating expenditures when they are currently well but seeking to anticipate future demand. Members cast their votes in accordance with their own perceptions of risk and some idea about the level of medical services they are likely to need in the future. Then the collective level of provision will depend on the preferences of members of the community; and if there is any divergence of preference, as there is bound to be, it will ultimately depend upon the voting rule that is used to amalgamate those preferences into a collective choice. I shall suppose (what is, in fact, embarrassingly controversial for the responsive model) that the collective choice is well formed, in the sense that there is a clear and definitive result from the voting procedure.[9] The result of the voting, then, yields a choice about the desired level of provision. Here, then, we have a clear statement of the community's willingness to pay for its own medical care. Can we not take this statement as the justification for the particular level of resources that are supplied, always supposing that the level of provision is in accordance with this expressed wish?

To see why not, consider that it is only in an *ersatz* sense that the voting procedure represents the community's willingness to pay for medical services. As long as there are diverse preferences about the level of services it is desirable to provide, there will always be some people for whom the agreed level of provision under-supplies their needs. Such people may be particularly risk averse, or they may be especially concerned about the quality of care, or they may simply be more farseeing than others about what real needs exist and be willing to anticipate future demands in their present expenditure. Now it may be argued at this point that it is this diversity of preference that provides the most cogent ground for permitting private provision alongside public provision, for in that way the needs of the most sensitive or concerned can be reflected in their willingness to supplement public provision with private insurance cover. But this is to neglect two important considerations. The first of these is that the divergence between a person's own assessment of a suitable level of care and the level of care provided as a result of community voting may well be substantial in a large number of cases. The logic of this situation is to make the public provision only a residual affair and to encourage individuals to take out suitable private cover for themselves. If it is responsiveness to preferences that we are worried about, markets are more likely to be successful want-regarding institutions than governments, and this to some extent will undermine the sense that it is the task of the government to make provision for the health care needs of the mass of citizens.

The second consideration is that any disposition to use markets must be tempered by the thought that, although markets respond to the willingness to pay, they do so only if there is an ability to pay, and it is just this lack of ability to pay that was one of the motives originally leading to a desire to suspend or attenuate market arrangements in the field of medical provision.

This might not be so much of a problem if it could be shown that there was an obvious authority and rightness about taking the decision of the community that emerged from the voting process as the community's level of provision, but there is unlikely to be any logical basis for this belief. The same set of preferences in a community amalgamated by a different voting rule will yield a different collective choice. For example, if the voting rule requires the collective outcome to secure not merely a simple majority but a qualified majority, then the same preferences will be translated into a quite distinct collective choice. There is not much sense to the notion that the result of a vote represents a community's willingness to pay for health care, if some other voting rule would have yielded quite distinct results.[10] The conclusion must therefore be that the responsive model of government is unsatisfactory as a basis on which to suppose that issues of health spending can be decided. We must turn instead to the model of responsible government.

## Responsible government

The model of responsible government operates on the assumption that the task of government is to justify a course of action rather than act as an amalgamation device for the preferences that exist. It must produce reasons for the policies that are adopted and these must be subject to public scrutiny. Politics, on this model, resembles a process of discussion rather than a process of voting. Instead of working with fixed preferences which are then amalgamated in some way to produce a collective choice, the concept of discussion involves an attempt to redefine and refine preferences in the light of public debate. The authority of responsible government comes from its ability to convince and persuade, rather than from a counting of the number of voices on one side and on the other.

The fundamental notion here is that of political accountability. As Day and Klein[11] have pointed out, the concept of accountability really has two distinct senses. The first of these is concerned with agents rendering an explanation or account of their actions in the light of an agreed purpose or set of purposes – for example, when organisations present financial accounts to show how monies have been spent. However, there is a second and broader sense of accountability: institutions are accountable when they have to justify to some relevant public the purposes they are pursuing. Accountability in this broader sense pertains to ends as well as means: a government is accountable when it can show that the policies it is pursuing are justified in the light of a public set of values.

If we reflect upon the requirements it is necessary to satisfy if a system of public accountability is to function effectively then we shall see that at least three conditions will be needed. The first of these may be termed the condition of publicity. This requires that decisions taken should be justifiable in a public fashion. Its most general use is to exclude private or partisan interests from asserting themselves in the process of policy making. For example, it is unlikely, given the condition of publicity, that a ruling party would seek to justify a course of action on the grounds that it was conducive to its own party advantage. The condition of publicity does not rule out such a reason being given – merely asserting that whatever reasons lay behind the decision should be publicly stated – but it is highly unlikely that any governing party would want to be seen pursuing policies whose main purpose was to promote a narrow party interest. So in this way the principle of publicity prevents decisions being made that are against the public interest.

The second condition is that accountability should be discharged in terms of the values that obtain within the political culture of the society in question. Since it is a question of justifying ends as well as means, the government will have to appeal to values embedded in the political culture in which its conduct is located. There is no assumption here that a political culture is simple or uncontentious. Indeed, quite the opposite. Political disagreements often arise because of varying inter-pretations of values within a political culture. However, the identity of a political community is in part defined by the content of its political culture, and this means that an accountable government will necessarily draw upon the terms of that culture in justifying its policy choices.

The third condition is that of honesty. Since the task of government is to persuade and convince, it will not be in a position to do so unless it treats issues honestly and openly. A public dialogue that is premissed on information available to all and on principles that are explicitly stated stands some chance of generating a consensus. A public dialogue in which the government withholds some crucial information or uses the public discussion as a front behind which the real decisions are taken cannot be expected to generate a consensus.

What relevance does this conception of government have for questions concerned with the allocation of scarce medical resources? Its chief relevance is to state the procedural conditions that a government needs to satisfy if it is to sustain the obligation of justifying its choices. In other words, the concept of responsible government places limits on the manner in which the government is able to make and present choices about the allocation of resources. It may help to see the force of the ideas being advanced if the practical implications they might be thought to have are considered. Although I have suggested that we cannot expect an argument in political philosophy to yield specific practical conclusions, it is equally true that procedural principles must set some limits on what may be tolerated by way of the principled use of power. And it is to a discussion of these potential practical applications that I now turn.

## Practical implications

According to the conception of democracy as the responsible exercise of political power, it is the task of the government to explain the basis on which it makes financial allocations to the provision of medical care. If the decision is an open and public one, then it ought to be possible for those making the decisions to state, even if in only broad terms, what standard and quality of care is implied by these financial allocations. This, in turn, means that the government should have a public view about the scope of provision and a set of standards for knowing when the quality of care is adequate for the clinical conditions that fall within the scope of its coverage.

In terms of the particular institutional arrangements of the NHS, this requirement is complicated by the fact that it is the health authorities, rather than the government itself, which are responsible for the provision of services. Nonetheless, since financial provision for the service is made by the government, a responsible policy would involve an explicitly stated view on the part of the Department of Health about the standards an efficient and well-administered authority should attain. For the major clinical conditions this would involve statistical standards concerned with waiting times, recovery rates and other quality of care indicators. The DOH would, in effect, be saying that for the allocated volume of resources the expectation is that the average authority should be able to provide a certain standard of care. By making explicit the implications of its allocation in this way, the government would be committing itself to revising its allocation or expectation if it could be shown that the putative standard of provision could not be attained at the existing level of resources.

Consider what this might mean in practice. There is no intrinsic reason why there should not be a public policy of withholding certain expensive drugs or clinical procedures from those who need them. It is a perfectly valid argument to say that their costs outweigh any conceivable benefits, or that the sacrifice of other goods, including the good of economic prosperity, would not be worth the outcome. What is not justifiable is to pretend that such drugs or procedures are available, or to present the issue as though no choice was being made. In other words, the concept of responsible government implies a degree of honesty and publicity in the decisions made on the allocation of resources.

The effect of this approach is to make the government provision of health care resemble a form of insurance. Just as insurers have to be explicit about the coverage they are prepared to give, so a responsible government would need to be explicit about the level and quality of care it thought appropriate to provide. The difference between the two, however, is that insurers are not expected to justify their position. They offer commercial terms, and those who want something better either find another insurer or they have to accept that no insurer finds it worthwhile entering that particular market. With publicly provided health care, by contrast, there is an expectation that the government will not only seek to justify its decision but will revise its financial allocation should public debate indicate that this is the reasonable course of action.

It might also be thought that by making the public finance of health care resemble an explicit form of insurance the government should be legally liable for any deficiencies in the provision of care. However, the Collier case shows that there is no legal right to health care in the form of a claim upon resources that the United Kingdom courts are prepared to uphold. The obligation of the health authorities and of the Secretary of State is to provide care to a level that is judged subjectively reasonable, and the courts will not insist that any other standard of provision is enforced. However, if we begin to think of the provision of health care explicitly on the model of insurance, it seems natural to question this state of affairs and wonder whether it should be allowed to continue; or whether, instead, UK citizens should have a right to a certain standard of care that would be legally and constitutionally upheld. There is (in my view at least) no easy answer to this issue.

There is something essentially unsatisfactory about a service which for most people is a monopoly supplier of what is, sometimes literally, a life-saving resource which remains free to determine whether treatment should be withheld in particular cases and which does not have to defend legally the resource decisions that are made. On the other hand, there is the danger that decisions about the allocation of resources will be distorted if citizens become able to pursue, through the courts, a right to treatment. Courts are, of course, only able to look at particular cases and by determining that a patient with a particular condition is entitled to treatment the courts may well provide an incentive on the part of administrators to ensure that certain conditions are well-provided for, giving less priority to rare or minority conditions where those who suffer may be less well-placed to pursue their claims. If 'defensive medicine' is an evil to be avoided, so is 'defensive health administration'.

From the point of view of the principles involved there is a difficult balance to be struck. My own tentative conclusion is that there are no grounds *a priori* for ruling out a legally enforceable entitlement to treatment under a scheme by which the government was made politically accountable for its resource allocations. Equally, however, any attempt to implement such a proposal ought to proceed cautiously with an eye to the problems that might arise.

One advantage of the government being explicit about its resource assumptions is that it creates the conditions for the pursuit of other desirable goals in the allocation of health care resources. Whatever the level of the total allocation, there will always be a need to ensure that resources are used efficiently and effectively. There is sufficient evidence to show that although standards of practice are, on average, high in British medicine, there are pockets of ineffective (and sometimes simply negligent) practice that are worrying to anyone concerned about the quality of patient care.[12] It will almost certainly take the introduction of some form of regular peer review to improve the situation. Yet there is the inevitable whiff of a double standard when a government insists on introducing greater accountability for those who work in the service without itself taking steps to ensure that it is itself accountable for the decisions within its power. If there were a greater willingness on the part of governments to ensure that their own decision-making was conducted responsibly, it should prove easier to make all the health professions more accountable.

## Conclusion

There is a persistent temptation, when considering the allocation of health care resources, to suppose that there is a mechanical solution to the problems involved. Such solutions are sometimes supposed to reside in a formula that will incorporate self-evident principles of fairness, or in a set of absolute requirements that ensure patients are not denied their rights. In contrast to this mechanical approach, the concept of responsible government presents something far less ambitious. If politics is seen on the model of discussion, then it will have the character of discussion. It will be open-textured, unpredictable and sometimes ambiguous. More importantly, policy making will be seen to be an activity in which the right answer is not something to be discovered, but something to be constructed as part of the common life that living in a society involves.

The challenge of health policy making is that as the discussion proceeds the problems are likely to become more serious rather than less. The rate of innovation in the development of health technologies is such that the cost pressures will increase, not decrease, over time. Moreover, as expectations rise about the quality of life that the mass of citizens can expect to enjoy, there is every reason to believe that the demand for a high standard of health care will grow. There is, then, no escape from the need for responsible decision making in this area.

Who will bear the burden of this decision making? I suggested at the beginning that the burden was wrongly placed if it fell upon individual physicians. To put physicians in a situation in which they must deceive their patients about the reasons for denying treatment is to strain their loyalties to the limit. On the other hand, we perhaps also ought to recognise that there is a burden here. The economic constraints on the availability of treatment are just as sharp as the technical ones. When patients are faced with a life-threatening or severe condition, they are likely to be weak and vulnerable. No matter how responsible the political system has been in making its decisions, clinicians will always have to cope with this weakness and vulnerability. At this point, right conduct ceases to be a property of institutions and becomes an aspiration of persons. No doubt there is an ethic that applies to that situation that will help practitioners avoid the evils of deception on the one hand and inhumanity on the other. But that must be the subject of another chapter.

## Notes and references

1  This is a stylised version of a real example more fully reported in Albert Weale (ed). Cost and choice in health care: the ethical dimension (Report prepared by a working party on the ethics of resource allocation in the health care system). London, King Edward's Hospital Fund for London, 1988, chapter 1.

2  See, among others, H Aaron and W B Schwartz. The painful prescription: rationing hospital care. Washington DC, The Brookings Institution, 1984; S Challah and others. Negative selection of patients for dialysis and transplantation in the United Kingdom. British Medical Journal, 288, 6424, pages 1119–1122; D Rennie and others. Limited resources and the treatment of end-stage renal failure in Britain and the United States. Quarterly Journal of Medicine NS, 56, 219, pages 321–336.

3  K J Arrow. Uncertainty and the welfare economics of medical care. American Economic Review, 53, 5, pages 941–973. For a good up-to-date summary of recent arguments see N Barr. The economics of the welfare state. London, Weidenfeld and Nicolson, 1987, pages 293–301.

4  Robert G Evans. The spurious dilemma: reconciling medical progress and cost control. Quarterly Journal of Health Service Management, 4, 1, pages 25–34.

5  Fritz Beske. Expenditures and attempts at cost containment in the statutory health insurance system of the Federal Republic of Germany. In: Gordon McLachlan and Alan Maynard (eds). The

public/private mix for health: the relevance and effects of change. London, Nuffield Provincial Hospitals Trust, 1982, pages 233–263.

6  This restriction to the 'basic structure' follows the tradition established by J Rawls. A theory of justice. Oxford, Clarendon Press, 1972, pages 7–11.

7  This conception of politics, which ultimately goes back to Aristotle, can be found in the writings of Hannah Arendt; for example, The human condition. Chicago, University of Chicago Press, 1958.

8  J Schumpeter. Capitalism, socialism and democracy. London, Allen and Unwin, 1954, page 285.

9  For a clear discussion of the problems which lurk in the mechanisms of preference amalgamation see W H Riker. Liberalism against populism. San Francisco, W H Freeman and Co, 1982. Riker illustrates the practical force of the crucial theoretical results with a brilliantly told series of stories in The art of political manipulation. New Haven, Yale University Press, 1986.

10 Compare W H Riker. Liberalism again populism, chapter 2 (see note 9 above).

11 P Day and R Klein. Accountabilities. London, Tavistock, 1987, chapter 1.

12 Accounting for perioperative deaths. The Lancet, 2, 8572, 1987, pages 1369–1371; John N Lunn and H Brendan Devlin. Lessons from the confidential enquiry into perioperative deaths in three NHS regions. The Lancet, 2, 8572, 1987, pages 1384–1386.

# AIDS and tolerance

## Richard Harries

Our society takes a wide degree of tolerance for granted. We
assume people are and will be basically tolerant, but this is a
highly dangerous attitude. History shows that people are not
fundamentally tolerant. Such tolerance as we now enjoy in the
areas of religion, race or sexuality has had to be fought for
fiercely and for a long time. Only just over 20 years ago
homosexual practice was a criminal offence. We certainly
cannot assume that the tolerance we now enjoy will continue
automatically. It could be that in the long tunnel of world
history it will have been a tiny candle which flickered for a few
years in certain parts of Europe and North America. If we want
it to burn longer than that we will have to cup our hands
around the flickering flame.

In order to safeguard and prolong a relatively tolerant
society it is necessary to look at the roots of intolerance. First,
there is our attitude to disease. It is not true that we have an
instinctive feeling of sympathy and pity for those who are sick.
This may be present, but we also view disease with a mixture of
ignorance, fear, disgust and hostility. As human beings we
react to one another first of all at a basically physical or, if you
like, chemical or biochemical level. We like or dislike the
colour of a person's hair or the shape of his nose, the outline
of his body, the colour of his skin or the look in his eyes.
This basic reaction at a physical level occurs in our relationships with members of the opposite sex and the same sex.
When there is some obvious manifestation of sickness or
abnormality this is recognised, registered and responded to at
the unconscious level. Teenagers know this all too well, hence
their self-consciousness about how they look and their pre-
occupation with such universal symptoms as acne or teenage

spots. Those with something different about them are also acutely conscious of this phenomenon. Mr Gorbachev, who has a prominent birthmark on his head, is apparently anxious to keep this covered up as much as possible in front of the television cameras. William Golding's novel, *Darkness Invisible*, has as its central character a strange man called Matty. Matty emerges mysteriously at the beginning of the book out of the London blitz, in which he had been badly burned and disfigured. As a young boy he lay in hospital being treated. Golding describes the reaction to him in the following words:

> In hospital, adults hurrying to their own unfortunates, were repelled by the sordid misery in which Matty passed his days, and they flashed sideways at him an uneasy smile which he interpreted with absolute precision.

Faced with disease, we wish at the least to avert our eyes and at the worst to push the diseased person away from us. We want to keep him out sight and out of mind. This is particularly so if we believe that the disease is contagious. The classic example in the Bible is leprosy, which was probably not what modern scientific medicine means by leprosy but was a word which indicated a wide range of skin diseases. Leviticus chapter 13, verses 42 to 46 reads:

> And if there be in the bald head, or bald forehead, a white reddish sore; it *is* a leprosy sprung up in his bald head, or his bald forehead. Then the priest shall look upon it: and, behold, *if* the rising of the sore *be* white reddish in his bald head, or in his bald forehead, as the leprosy appeareth in the skin of the flesh; He is a leprose man, he *is* unclean: the priest shall pronounce him utterly unclean; his plague *is* in his head. And the leper in whom the plague *is*, his clothes shall be rent, and his head bare, and he shall put a covering upon his upper lip, and shall cry, Unclean, unclean. All the days wherein the plague *shall be* in him he shall be defiled; he *is* unclean: he shall dwell alone; without the camp *shall* his habitation *be*.

There is a further factor as far as those with AIDS are concerned. For not only will they develop various abrasions on the skin they are, at the present stage of medical knowledge, dying. This raises the question of our attitude not only to disease but to death. Death, like illness or disfigurement, is a spectre from which we seek to avert our eyes or shut away out of sight.

One piece of wisdom that this century has sought to learn afresh is the value of facing our feelings, of being honest about what we feel and think. Sometimes this wisdom has gone along with a piece of unwisdom – namely, that feelings once faced should then be automatically acted out in the interest of an unrepressed and fulfilled self. But this unwisdom does not at all necessarily follow on from the wisdom of facing what we feel. Freud, above all, alerted us to the fact that whatever we consciously think or say we may at the unconscious level be responding in a very different way. Furthermore, if there are aspects of response that have not been taken into consciousness they may, though repressed, be active in dangerous forms of projection. The result is that we attribute to other people aspects of ourself that we have not come to terms with or fear in others what we fear to discover in ourselves.

In facing disease and death people must find help from where they can. However, for those who are so minded, there are resources within the Christian tradition which can undoubtedly help. First, there is the biblical view that we are clay, dust, mortal flesh and blood. On Ash Wednesday many Christians have a piece of ash put on their foreheads with the words: 'Remember O man that thou art dust and to dust thou shalt return'. We share with the most diseased person a common flesh and blood, a common mortality. Secondly, however much we are of the earth, this dust, this clay, has been breathed into by the living spirit of God. We have been stamped with the divine image and have the capacity to reflect His glory and share His immortality. The result is that when a Christian faces an old person who is incontinent and senile, or someone who is schizophrenic, or someone suffering from Down's syndrome, he will be conscious of relating to a living soul. If we needed any reminder of this we have had recent eloquent testimony in the award of the Whitbread prize for literature to Christy Nolan for his novel *Under the Eye of the Clock*. Christy Nolan, as you know, has been totally paralysed from birth, unable to speak or move.

The result is that the Christian faith at its best has inspired the followers of Jesus to an uncompromising affirmation of the eternal worth of those whom society instinctively wishes to push outside the camp. Whether at the personal level, symbolised by St Francis kissing the leper, or Father Damien spending his ministry on a leper island until he too caught leprosy, or the work of Mother Teresa among the dying destitutes of the streets of Calcutta, the deeper resources in which true tolerance must be rooted have been revealed.

Sidney Carter once wrote a short poem based on a poster depicting Mother Teresa bending over an emaciated body, perhaps cutting the man's finger nails. It reads:

*Your Levity*

No revolution will come in time
to alter this man's life,
except the one surprise of being loved.

He has no interest in civil rights,
neo-Marxism,
psychiatry, or any kind of sex.

He has only twelve more hours to live,
so never mind about
a cure for cancer, smoking, leprosy,
or osteo-arthritis.

Over this dead loss to society
you pour your precious ointment,
call the bluff,
and laugh at the fat and clock-faced gravity
of our economy.
You wash the feet that will not walk tomorrow.

Come, levity of love
show him; show me,
in this last step of time
Eternity, leaping and capering.

Whether Christian or not, however, we need to find such help as we can in order to face as honestly as possible our own feelings about disease and death and to find a vision to affirm the unique value of each person, whatever state they are in or whatever stage of life they have reached. As far as AIDS is concerned, however, there is another factor. For we are here dealing with people who are not only diseased and dying but are associated in the public mind predominantly with homosexuality. Although, as we know, in Africa AIDS is primarily a disease among heterosexuals, in Europe and North America it has until now been largely confined to the homosexual community. The November 1987 figures of people with AIDS/HIV in the United Kingdom are as follows:

1170 (665 of whom are dead) including –
  986 gay/bisexual men
  43 heterosexuals
  17 drug users
  68 people with haemophilia
  16 blood recipients who received their blood abroad
   8 blood recipients who received their blood in the UK
  13 children of AB+ mothers
   2 undetermined

At the recent International Conference on AIDS Prevention, Everett Koop, Surgeon General of the United States, pointed out that although the number of heterosexual victims is growing, both as a proportion and as an absolute number, only four per cent of American AIDS victims are heterosexual and, he claimed, there is little likelihood of an AIDS explosion among heterosexuals in western nations. Instead the west faces the prospect of a 'leakage' into mainstream society which could prove difficult to contain. If this is so, then AIDS is likely to continue to be associated in the public mind in Europe and North America with homosexuality. I began by pointing out that the tolerance we enjoy in our society has been short lived. And of nothing is this more true than in our attitude towards homosexuality, which until 20 years ago was a criminal offence. A good indication of how things were before the 1967 Wolfenden report, and therefore how a good many people in our society still feel, can be gained by consideration of Tennessee Williams' play *Cat on a Hot Tin Roof*. The tension of the play revolves around the fact that Brick has enjoyed a close friendship with a college friend, which he idealises as something wonderful, but which he fears other people will suspect of being homosexual. At one point Brick says to his wife Maggie:

One man has one great good true thing in his life, one great good thing which is true! I had friendship with Skippe. You are naming it dirty.

A useful contrast can be made between that play, which was written in 1955, and the example of homosexuality in the film *My Beautiful Laundrette*. As *The Independent* pointed out in a leader, homosexuals believe that homosexuality itself, rather than a sexually transmitted disease, is now on trial after 20 years of toleration in this country. In recent months we have seen the debate at the General Synod of the Church of England, where the Synod took a much firmer line against homosexual practice than it has done for the last 20 years; the resignation of a judge as a result of letters revealing a homosexual relationship; and, most seriously of all, Clause 28 of the Local Government Bill. This, as originally framed, would make it a crime to promote homosexuality in schools. Even the amendment brought about by opposition to Clause 28 is worrying. There is grave danger that homophobia, fanned by some quarters in the popular press, will take over.

Another piece of wisdom we have tried to learn this century, wisdom associated primarily with Jung rather than Freud, is that there is a spectrum of sexuality and that we all share both masculine and feminine characteristics. This is not to say that no distinction can be made between a heterosexual and a homosexual person. As Dr Johnson said, the fact of twilight does not obliterate the distinction between night and day. However, there will be aspects in all of us that are attracted to, in the widest sense of the word, members of the same sex as well as members of the opposite sex. This is another fact that has to be faced at the personal and not simply the general level. Here, the dangers of repression leading to projection can be especially dangerous. In earlier generations there really were witch hunts. Whole communities could become hysterically concerned to eliminate all those with the slightest taint of witchcraft from their midst. Arthur Miller wrote about such a community in *The Witches of Salem*. We have to remember, too, that in Nazi Germany not only Jews but members of other minority groups – gypsies, mental defectives and homosexuals – were harried and put to death.

The formation of our identity as persons involves overlapping psychological, social and theological considerations. At the psychological level, prejudice and intolerance are defences which enable us to maintain our own sense of worth by projecting our unacknowledged and undesirable characteristics onto those we label inferior or evil. This is undoubtedly happening in the AIDS crisis. By this mechanism a person is able to see all the badness in the other rather than in themselves; and to fight it in 'the enemy' or 'the heretic' rather than in themselves. The Christian faith has matters of supreme import to offer to this situation; that our worth is not identical with that part of ourselves we approve of. Rather, as Luther said, we are *simul iustus et peccator* – at once unacceptable and utterly accepted. Our value is to be found in our totality as a person, not by splitting off an allegedly good part from an allegedly bad part.

Social psychologists suggest that we find our identity as people by identifying with the mores and outlook of the groups to which we belong and that those groups find their character by contrasting themselves with other groups. So the English tell stories about the Scots and Irish and *vice versa*, thereby reinforcing their solidarity with the group and their own identity at the same time. This seems to be an inevitable and not totally to be rejected part of growing into identity. So those who come to King's College London, having failed to obtain a place at Oxbridge, rapidly develop a proper sense of the superiority of all education at London University, compared to Oxford or Cambridge. Those who have had the good fortune to be accepted at King's College contrast themselves favourably with those at University College. Much of this is relatively harmless and part of the process of finding ourselves. But it turns nasty when it is directed against the weak and vulnerable or when there are strong forces of prejudice around waiting for a socially acceptable outlet, as has for so much of the time been true of attitudes to Jews. Again, Christian theology seems to have something important to say. Our identity is to be found not in contrast to the allegedly negative characteristics of members of other groups but through what we share with them – our common humanity, morality and, above all, our brokenness – if not now at least in the hour of our death. We belong with others and find our identity in communion with them, not apart from others and in contrast to them. Jesus called into the community all manner of disreputables and ne'er-do-wells. The first Christians called this motley fellowship the body or very self of Christ. For the Christian this truth is particularly poignant, in relation to those who are dying of AIDS. For some will be fellow believers within the body of Christ.

At the heart of a belief in tolerance is a profound respect for individual liberty. We may believe a person to be mistaken in his beliefs and misguided in his life-style. Nevertheless, we will want to afford him the maximum freedom to control his own destiny and we will challenge all that seeks to restrict that freedom. Some people may believe in tolerance because they think that one set of beliefs is as good as another and no particular life-style should be classed as superior to any other. On this view the state and the main institutions of society are morally neutral. This is not my view. There is no space to develop the point, but suffice it to say that I do not believe that anything can be morally neutral. Every institution, whether it likes it or not, expresses a certain set of values and assumptions. My point would be, that among this set of values and assumptions, there should be the highest possible affirmation of personal liberty. Not moral indifferentism but a moral vision which includes a profound respect for personal choice is the foundation of toleration.

It will be argued by some that there are certain situations of national emergency when personal liberties can and must be curtailed. This is quite correct. Personal liberty is not absolute. In wartime, for example, personal freedoms are restricted in many ways. Similarly, if there is a national epidemic it would be quite right to curtail certain personal freedoms. But in making out a case for such restriction it is possible to see why a case *cannot* be made out at the present time in relation to the threat of AIDS. Let us make out a case for the restriction of personal freedom. Suppose, for example, there was a particularly virulent form of flu and this was spread very quickly and easily simply by inhaling air into which someone else had sneezed or coughed. Moreover, this flu virus led within three years to irreversible brain damage and premature senility. It would not take a fascist to see that in such a terrible situation there would have to be mass screening and quarantining. However, to posit that example is to reveal how far from that kind of situation we are even with the terrible threat of AIDS. AIDS is not spread simply by breathing in air. It is spread through certain clearly known and avoidable activities, particularly anal intercourse and injection with needles that have been used by other drug users. Equally, the way to avoid any risk of AIDS is equally well known. It is true that there is still some slight risk, for example, through receiving a transfusion of contaminated blood. However, steps have been taken and are being taken to rather reduce such risks to the bare minimum. Furthermore, screening people for AIDS is not an effective test. What screening can reveal is the presence of antibodies contacted four months or more before the time of the test. Such tests cannot reveal the presence of HIV that has been contacted in the four months immediately before the test. So a negative test could do actual harm in that it might induce false confidence.

Of course, the strictest precautions should be taken in all situations where there is contact with blood – in operating theatres, for example; and the strictest standards already prevail there. To go further and seek through screening and quarantining to isolate HIV carriers would be a gross infringement of personal liberties with no substantial benefit to society as a whole. It would be pandering to a deep seated but impossible-to-fulfil human desire: the desire for a risk-free society. Part of the contribution that religion should make is that it helps society to live with an unavoidable element of risk without getting in a panic and focusing on scapegoats.

Tolerance seems a somewhat weak word and a wimpish idea. However, if our society is to continue to be a relatively tolerant one a great deal of strength will be required. People sometimes think of tolerance in terms of 'live and let live'. This is a totally inadequate notion for the simple reason that other people's lives impinge upon me and my living impinges upon them. We do not, for the most part, live in self-contained compartments isolated from one another. It is interesting that the root of the Latin word from which tolerance is derived, *tolerare*, means 'to bear'. Tolerance, therefore, means bearing with or putting up with a certain amount of irritation, discomfort or hurt within oneself rather than suppressing the activities of other people in order to avoid irritation, discomfort or hurt. This has at least two aspects to it, the first of which is an instinctive tendency to moralise and blame other people. AIDS victims are particularly liable to become the object of moral censoriousness and Christians will want to bear in mind two sayings of Jesus: 'Judge not that ye be not judged' and 'Forgive us our sins as we forgive those who sin against us'. Also, St Paul wrote: 'for there is no difference: For all have sinned and come short of the glory of God' (Romans chapter 3, verses 22–23). There is no reason to think that AIDS victims or HIV carriers have fallen short in any more morally culpable way than the rest of us.

Secondly, and more positively, having overcome the instinctive tendency to blame, there is the obligation to help and support one another. Another text comes to mind: 'Bear ye one another's burdens and so fulfil the law of Christ' (Galatians chapter 6, verse 2). And this does seem to be happening in the homosexual community. People are not only adjusting their life-styles, they are supporting one another at a personal level and raising funds to support the sick at an institutional level. Ian McKellan, through donating the proceeds of his one man performance of Shakespeare, has personally raised nearly £500,000 for the London Lighthouse Project which has been set up to help AIDS victims. When I spoke to one of the people behind that project in the early stages he surprised me by saying that what it had to offer was real gospel. I was surprised because I know that this friend, though religious, certainly does not force what he believes down the throats of others. But what he meant was that through ministering to AIDS victims, helping them to face up to their condition and making the most of the time that was left to them, there had so often come about a real increase in the quality of their lives. Life had suddenly begun to have, for quite a number, a sense of its preciousness, intensity, quality and mutual caring.

The Diocese of Oxford has brought out a booklet on AIDS, which is I venture to suggest one of the best productions yet. In addition to a chapter on the basic facts about AIDS, it has a chapter of theological reflection and a final chapter on the pastoral dimension. This was written by a nun who has spent much of her ministry working with AIDS victims in America. She movingly describes how much is to be received from those suffering from AIDS as well as what can be given to them.

In this we see something of the true meaning of tolerance: not simply living and letting live but a mutual giving and receiving in our common suffering and mortality.

# The ethics of sex selection

John Mahoney

When the first successful results of *in vitro* fertilisation began to appear, Dr Robert Edwards complained that scientists had for years been asking the philosophers, the moralists and the churches to address the ethical aspects of IVF and that they had not done so. In what he said Dr Edwards was mistaken; but in what he meant, or implied, he was correct. There had for years been articles on the ethics and implications of IVF – treated seriously in various journals and with varying degrees of science-fiction alarm in the Sunday press. But even though there was a growing body of writing on the subject there was no ethical consensus emerging on IVF in those days, any more than there is today. And that was what Dr Edwards really appeared to want: agreed ethical guidance for the doctors, scientists and patients involved in developing and applying this dramatic new procedure for treating human infertility.

The possibility of the sex selection of children – of predetermining the gender of a child – is today just beginning to appear over the horizon and informed discussion on the ethical aspects and implications is still rather rare and scattered. But the consequences of such an innovation are, in my view, likely to be much more profound and far-reaching for society than the implications of IVF. And, I would hazard a guess, once society realises that it is becoming possible to select the sex of children, the resulting debate and controversy will far outstrip current debates on IVF, surrogacy and embryo-experimentation.

It would be diverting to predict the positions and stances likely to be adopted by various groups in society: the tabloid newspapers, the royal colleges, the various religious bodies, and the government. However, for my present purposes I wish simply to adopt a sort of 'early-warning' attitude to the whole question – not in any alarmist sense, far less in the sense of offering firm moral answers to the questions which the subject inevitably raises. What I propose is the more modest, but more constructive, approach of aiming to identify at this early stage what are the moral issues involved in the sex selection of children and to offer some reflections on these issues.

I propose to address the subject progressively. I begin by considering the techniques and procedures involved in sex selection; move then to consider the possible effects on the children who thus result; then the motivation of the potential parents who choose to adopt the procedure; and finally the wider implications for society as a whole which might result from sex selection of children becoming easily and generally available.

It is already possible to identify whether an existing fetus is male or female by ultrasound scanning or amniocentesis at about the 16th week of pregnancy. Another method, at an earlier stage of pregnancy, is chorion biopsy, where membrane is abstracted from the fetal sac and examined for its chromosomal structure. And there are also attempts being made at sexual identification at the earliest stages of *in vitro* fertilisation. In Italy, for example, the technique of embryo biopsy is used whereby a cell is removed to ascertain the embryo's genetic structure before introducing the embryo into the womb if it meets requirements. But what is envisaged in sex *selection* takes place before conception. In Japan, for example, centrifugation is used on the collected male sperm to differentiate the sex-determining X and Y chromosomes prior to using the selected sperm in IVF or in artificial insemination.

Such methods of sex determination rely heavily on technology and skilled intervention and their application is, therefore, comparatively infrequent. What is foreseen, however, is the development of simpler and more widely available methods of selection at the pre-conception stage – by recourse, for example, to pills or a diaphragm to differentiate between the semen bearing the X and Y chromosomes (as already achieved in the laboratory through the use of a centrifuge). By this means, sex selection will be brought within easy reach of all couples in society who wish to take advantage of it without the need to have recourse to infanticide, to gender abortion after amniocentesis or chorion biopsy, or to *in vitro* fertilisation.

It is readily understandable that those who are morally opposed to infanticide, or abortion, or the discarding of embryos as a matter of principle, will be equally opposed to their use as a means to avoid having a child of what is considered the 'wrong' sex. It is equally understandable that those who are morally opposed in principle to artificial insemination will logically resist the application of this practice to predetermine the sex of a child. Such objections would not apply, however, to preselecting the sex of a child by the use of diaphragms or pills before or at the time of normal intercourse and fertilisation. And even individuals, or bodies such as the Roman Catholic Church, who are fundamentally opposed to any form of contraception could not, it appears, morally object to these last methods of sex preselection. For they are not contraceptive either in intent or in effect. They are not designed to prevent conception but to direct it in a certain manner. Their purpose and use is to achieve conception and to produce a child, albeit conception of a particular kind and a child of chosen or predetermined sex.

It appears, then, that when it becomes a general possibility for any couple to programme a future conception and make it sex-specific, if I may so express it, ethical objections must be sought elsewhere than in the moral evaluation of the means chosen to bring this about. But there are, perhaps, more fundamental questions below the surface of particular ways and means: questions about human attitudes to technology and, in this case, about the application of technology to the primordial human phenomenon of parenting. Such questions find regular expression from time to time in misgivings or accusations of 'tampering with nature' or, in more religious terms, of 'playing at God'. Sex preselection thus raises from a fresh perspective fundamental questions about how we regard our species in its evolutionary development, and of how interventionist or participatory our attitude is, or may be, to that development. Within the religious perspective the same questions are expressed in terms of humanity's moral responsibility to its divine creator, and to what degree God has, or has not, delegated to human creatures a share in the divine initiative and in divine providence.

Perhaps, however, one aspect of these questions is particularly highlighted by the possibility of sex preselection – what religious believers would call divine providence, and others would call simple chance or spontaneity. It is true that treatment for infertility already raises these questions of whether it is better for couples who have difficulty in procreating to leave the chances of having a child to nature or to God, and to accept the outcome with human resignation or religious trust. But I think that the more precise question, not of contriving to have a child but of contriving to have a boy or a girl, puts into sharper relief whether we are as individuals or as a species fundamentally better off when we are disposed to accept the normal, possibly random, processes of mother nature or, speaking religiously, are content to entrust such matters to God.

My intention here is not to attempt any detailed answer to these questions, but mainly to uncover them. I may permit myself, however, the personal observation that in Jewish and Christian religious terms the human calling to a stewardship of creation, whether the continuing co-creation of ourselves or of our environment, must entail some measure of personal and collective responsible initiative and of constructive adaptation to that environment. For in the normal human perspective, appealing to 'nature' (whether or not it is the product of divine activity and the agent of God's purpose) as a moral norm or guideline, is notoriously ambiguous. On the one hand, while the human scientific enterprise may be considered in many respects unnatural, in the sense of becoming increasingly artificial, this is because it at times finds nature, or the course of nature, seriously deficient in its structure and manifestations, and devotes much of its energy and other resources to remedying these deficiencies. And on the other hand, it is surely an important part of human nature to be intelligent, inventive and even manipulative, not only in evolutionary terms of survival but in religious terms of having been made in the image of an intelligent and enterprising God in order to continue his handiwork. Appeals, then, to the course of nature or to divine providence, I conclude, may be helpful as a last, perhaps resigned, resort, or when nothing else can be done. But it is a misunderstanding of nature in general, and an impoverishment and depreciation of human nature in particular, to invoke them as a moral veto on human action. We must look elsewhere for ethical criteria for our actions, and in this case for our attitude to preselecting the sex of future children.

This brings me to consider my second point: that of the interests of the child who results from the parental choice of his or her gender. There are some medical situations where it would clearly be of benefit for a child to be preselected in terms of sex. For instance, with genetic disorders and illnesses which are sex-connected, such as haemophilia and Duchenne muscular dystrophy, where normally only males are victims although females may be carriers. In such cases, the medical advantages for children of preselecting them for sex are obvious and need no further comment.

There is the additional consideration that the ability to preselect children for sex would not only significantly diminish the incidence of genetically inherited maladies, it could also, at a stroke, decrease the number of abortions in society. Sex preselection would thus render unnecessary the abortion on medical grounds of fetuses identified in the womb through chorion biopsy or amniocentesis as having sex-linked diseases. In a non-medical context, it would also remove the reason for gender-abortions of female fetuses which is done for social reasons in some ethnic communities in Britain and is developing on quite a large scale in some parts of India. It would also render unnecessary what is reported as happening in China, where the attempt to impose a social policy of one-child families results in the killing of baby girls at birth.

I may add, in passing, that some of the hostile public reaction to the revelation of gender-abortions in some ethnic communities in Britain on the grounds of social pressure (such as the prohibitive expense of dowries for marriageable girls) betrays, in my view, an obvious inconsistency which is at best muddle-headed, at worst hypocritical, and possibly even tinged with racism. For, if abortion is legal in Britain on the grounds of serious social pressure (although I do not myself consider it morally justified) then it is entirely logical to have recourse to it whatever the social or ethnic environment which produces and occasions that pressure. Much more so, as some commentators have pointed out, than the sometimes trivial reasons in the culture to which we are more accustomed which are permitted to masquerade, or are colluded in, as the social grounds for abortion envisaged by law.

To return to my main theme. If sex preselection of children were generally available this would certainly decrease the number of lives destroyed by abortion and this positive benefit would have to be balanced by the objection that sex-determined children were the result of deliberate human quality-control, with, it is claimed, a consequent diminution in their intrinsic humanity and personhood. This is already, of course, a basic objection by some people to the whole idea of artificial reproduction in general – that it treats the offspring as a 'product' to be tailored to other people's requirements. And once again the precision introduced by the idea, not just of whether or how to have a child by artificial procreation but of whether or how to have a girl or a boy, brings into greater prominence the question of the human control and the detailed specification of human reproduction.

In general I find no difficulty in rejecting the idea that artificial reproduction inevitably turns the resulting children into products of an inferior human status to their parents or to other children, for it can be counter-argued that children conceived by the last-resort and laborious process of IVF, to otherwise infertile couples, are likely to be very much wanted and cherished. But the same consideration cannot automatically be applied to children chosen to be boys or girls through manipulation of the embryo *in vitro* or through simple artificial insemination; far less to those children born as the result of popular easy methods of sex preselection. And it is here, then, that we need to consider the third point: the motivation of the parents in the choices they make.

It would no doubt be easy enough to see parental wish to have a boy or a girl in terms of simply satisfying the desires or needs of the future father and/or mother or of others in the family. There is, for instance, what might be called the 'son and heir' syndrome – the desire for a boy who will carry on the family, or rather the father's name, and inherit the family property or perhaps the family title. There might also be the desire for a daughter to become, in time, a congenial companion for the mother. And there might also be the wish for one or more child of both sexes in order to produce a nicely balanced family.

Moreover, boys might be considered desirable in order to provide for their parents in their old age, whereas daughters could be useful in looking after such elderly parents. (I shall return later to the possible sexist implications of all these remarks.)

Other possible parental motives for the sex selection of children could no doubt be identified. But the main ethical consideration in all of them appears to be this: are these desires for what we might call family engineering selfishly motivated, so as to be seen simply as potential parents using children to satisfy their own whims or desires or human needs? That seems to me to be altogether too cerebral and analytical an approach, and one which does not make due allowance for the normal human phenomenon of mixed motives. In many of our moral choices a primary consideration may be, and often is, accompanied by several other attractive features. And while these additional, or secondary, attractions might not be compelling in themselves, they can nevertheless contribute to a total bundle of human motivation for a particular choice and action, without dislodging the primary motive.

Moreover, apart from the medical advantages already mentioned, it could be a distinct personal and social advantage to be born a boy in some families or a girl in others. A girl, or another girl, might be particularly welcomed into a family totally or predominantly composed of brothers; a boy might be warmly received into a family of sisters. A boy born somewhere in the north of England might eventually receive the supreme accolade of being selected to play for Yorkshire County Cricket Club! A girl might find it particularly beneficial not to be expected to become a surrogate international rugby player for a frustrated father! More seriously, however, what these considerations bring to light is that parental motivation in the choice of sex for their children has to be seen not simply in terms of the satisfaction of individual needs or of the benefits to individuals, whether parents or children. That motivation has to be considered in terms of transmitting the gift of life and in terms of the family and the human community which is in the process of creation by the parents. Theirs is a heavy moral responsibility in deciding just to have a child, whatever its sex. And they are necessarily determining its genetic constitution, its environment, its character and its entire future by the unavoidable choices they make, whether consciously or not: the choice to have a child, the choice to do so in a particular country or town or climate, the choice to send it to a particular school, and the choice to encourage it or discourage it in certain forms of behaviour. Parenting is the pursuit of a series of choices which simply must be made, whether explicitly or implicitly. And inevitably these choices will mould a child. Some would see such choices, or some of them, as social indoctrination or as the packaging of a product. I prefer to view them as stages in the process of human procreation. And I do not see why, within such a chain of choices, the choice of sex should be singled out for particular moral disapproval.

But what happens if things go wrong? If the desired or expected boy turns out to be a girl, or vice versa? In my youth I was somewhat struck by a rather cloying novel entitled *Paddy, the Next Best Thing*, the story of a girl born to parents who had very much wanted a boy, but who just had to decide, when a girl arrived instead, to make the best of a bad job. I am not referring here to the question of gender assignment or gender identity in children, though that might not be irrelevant. What I have in mind is the moral risk of genetic abortion in the event of parental disappointment, or the subsequent emotional consequences for a child who came to discover and realise she or he had been born a disappointment to the parents. No doubt this already occurs in families where the parents simply hope for a boy or a girl without being able to do anything about it. But it would scarcely be surprising if the disappointment, or perhaps even the resentment, were the greater in those families where a couple had taken active steps to try to ensure the sex of their offspring. (The possible litigation against drug or medical supply companies for product-failure does not bear thinking about.)

Perhaps, again, this is overstating the case. There may be parallels with the cases of couples who, in spite of not wanting to have a child, or in spite of having taken precautions to avoid having one, find themselves faced with an unexpected or unwanted pregnancy. For it does not automatically follow, as is generally recognised as a matter of experience, that an unwanted pregnancy means an unwanted child. It happens that parents adjust in such cases, recover from the surprise or shock, and come positively to welcome and love the child for its own sake.

To sum up on this point of parental motivation: what all
these considerations might together indicate is the value and
desirability of counselling to any couple contemplating the
deliberate choice to have a child of a particular sex. Where there
are medical factors there is already provision for genetic
counselling, and now the range of choices would be much
more positive as a result of sex preselection techniques. But
there is much to be said also for the need for social counselling
to parents considering the sex-choice of their children, in order
to help them explore and evaluate their motivation and the
interests of the child. I conclude, however, that any couple
deciding to have a child are already deciding to determine its
human and personal characteristics through its genes and the
family and social environment into which it is going to be born.
It does not seem to me incontrovertibly wrong to aim to give
further explicit specification to that inheritance and environment by choosing whether it shall be a boy or a girl. And
indeed there are various positive reasons, as I have outlined,
which would lead to the conclusion that it could be positively
beneficial, and morally desirable, so to choose in individual
cases.

But, of course, we are not dealing simply with individual cases.
And that brings me to the final factor in assessing the ethics of
sex preselection in children: the overall social consequences of
such a practice being widely resorted to and the effects of such
a policy on society as a whole. It is a factor I find intriguing,
particularly when considering the pronouncements and views
of various bodies and individuals on the subject.
    The major misgiving expressed is that such a facility offered
to parents might lead to an undesirable imbalance of the sexes
in society. This was the view expressed, for instance, in the
report of the Working Party of the Council for Science and
Society on Human Procreation, against the background of its
'general impression that, in the long term, a society benefits
from having a roughly equal number of men and women'. And
these considerations led the Working Party to recommend
that, apart from medically desirable cases, 'sex should not be an
allowable factor in the selection of embryos for implanting in
the mother'.[1]
Interestingly, however, the government-sponsored Warnock

report was less confident on the undesirable social consequences if the sex selection of children became widely
available to couples. It foresaw the possibility in the not
too distant future of a reliable and simple method being
developed to select the sex of a child before fertilisation, even
on a 'do-it-yourself' basis; and it was dubious for several
reasons about the use of sex selection techniques on a wide
scale. But it found it impossible to predict the social consequences; and so it contented itself with suggesting that the
whole question of the acceptability of sex selection be kept
under review by the statutory licensing authority which it
suggested should be appointed.[2]

The White Paper, *Human Fertilisation and Embryology*,
currently under consideration with a view to Parliamentary
legislation and based substantially on the Warnock report,
does not refer explicitly to sex selection, though its provisions
for embryo research may be considered to cover the possibility
of sex selection on medical grounds as a result of embryo
biopsy. Therefore, if embryo research were permitted in law,
this could include projects aimed at advancing diagnostic or
therapeutic techniques or fertility control. And possibly this
could be taken to include sex identification of the early embryo
through biopsy in cases of suspected genetic sex-linked
diseases, with a view to implanting or rejecting the embryo
depending on the results of the test. And even if such research
were prohibited by a future law this may not outlaw procedures to ascertain the suitability of an embryo for transfer to
a woman's uterus or allowing an embryo to perish if an
abnormality is detected.[3] It appears however, as it stands, that
if the forthcoming legislation will outlaw sex selection of
children at the embryo stage or earlier on other than medical
grounds, it will do so only by implication.

But there is one particular sector of society which has
distinct and very explicit reservations about the social implications of the sex selection of children, and that is the sector
broadly identified as representing the women's movement.
The Warnock report observed that it is impossible to predict,
either in the long or the short term, the ratio of males to females
in society which might result from widespread sex selection.
But it recorded the suggestion that most couples would wish
their firstborn to be a boy, with the possible consequences of

his enjoying certain advantages over any sisters and with wider social implications for the role of women in society.[4] First a boy and then a girl would be the normal pattern, many feminists suggest; and this may well be the case in society at present. If so, such writers conclude, this will only serve to entrench and confirm the sexual stereotype and injustice, going as far back as Aristotle in the west, which considers females to be second-class human beings.

It is not, then, simply that sex choice would affect the sex ratio in society in favour of men, though it would probably do that; it is also, and perhaps primarily, that in the widespread preference for male firstborns, females will come to realise that 'they are chosen to be second', with what are described as incalculable psychological ramifications for such 'little sisters'.[5] And it is in this context that Helen Holmes and Betty Hoskins observe of the technology of making sex choices that 'the real heart of the problem is that sex choice technologies would nurture patriarchy'.[6]

But it is not only women who might suffer psychologically and by comparison as a result of popular sex selection. Clifford Longley wrote an article in *The Times* called 'Making the Best of Celibacy'. He began it by observing that 'an excess of men over women in the population in future means that many males growing up now may never marry, and they will be forced to learn how to defy the received wisdom that life without sex is unhealthy'. It will be necessary, he continued, to establish 'a positive value for the single lifestyle ... [otherwise] ... the future surplus of men over women will produce a group of dissatisfied and frustrated unmarried men, having little stake in, or care for, the welfare of others'.[7] Interestingly, he did not refer to the fact that such a dilemma has for long been a fact of life for many women in society.

Are all these various considerations, and others, of the possible social effects of cumulative sex preselection sufficient to provide some ethical guidance on how the possibility of sex preselection is to be received and applied by individuals in society? If it will result in an increased disparity in the numbers of males and females perhaps there is something to be learned from previous occurrences of such a phenomenon in history. For instance, the social consequences of the decreasing incidence of maternal deaths in childbirth, or of the waves of migration out of Europe and into North America and Australia, or particularly in the demographic consequences of war. The First World War, for instance, resulted in the deaths of ten million young men in Europe, and this led in England to what David Thomson describes as much vague postwar discussion of the 'surplus women' problem, which was to a large extent a 'deficit of men' problem.[8] Yet this was not to last; and various demographers comment on what Reinhard in his *Histoire de la Population Mondiale* calls the 'curious fact' that after the war the proportion of male births grew in Germany, England and France as if to reduce the consequences of the heavy male death rate during the war.[9]

However the phenomenon is explained, it appears as if previous disparities in the sex ratio in a given society proved to be temporary and tended to diminish or to right themselves once the initial cause or causes had passed. Would this, however, continue to be the case once a reliable method of sex preselection were made generally and permanently available? Apart from tragic or catastrophic disasters, any corrective which was considered necessary would need at least to include the element of deliberate choice to reverse the trend. Singer and Wells, for instance, invoke what seems very like a law of supply and demand when they suggest that 'the value placed on daughters might rise'.[10] But in general, or before that new market trend emerges, what weight is to be given to forecasts of an unbalanced sex ratio in society, or to feminist fears of increased sex discrimination, and what ethical conclusions can be drawn from them if they are accurate? There would be no little irony if a movement which makes so much of a woman's right to choose were to prohibit her freedom of choice in this area. And possibly it would be equally inhuman to advocate that women should deliberately choose to have daughters, or daughters first, simply as an anti-discriminatory move, since this would come perilously close to using children as a means to be used to further political or social ends.

Perhaps what needs to be questioned here is the extent to which society itself will change in its thinking and its attitudes when sex preselection becomes a real universal possibility, and when for the first time couples are faced with examining not just their hopes but their precise motives and presuppositions in the deliberate choice they are contemplating. Perhaps also it is useful to take into account the likelihood that sex selection will result in a decline in the total birthrate, as the phenomenon vanishes of some couples producing several children of one sex before finally having the boy or the girl they want. In commenting on the 'deficit of men' after the First World War, Thomson also drew attention to another effect in Britain which was perhaps not unconnected with the absence of men at the front or with the massive male mortality rate. This was the acceleration in the emancipation of women as they entered into the national war effort, and as a tide of social recognition built up which could not be reversed in the postwar period.[11] Is it too fanciful to suggest the parallel that if sex selection results in a significant overall reduction of the total pool of people to perform the varied social functions and tasks required for society to operate successfully, then sex differences will become increasingly irrelevant in public life, particularly since traditional sex roles are already breaking down, and despite any initial family disadvantage in childhood which might still be suffered by its female members? Yet, however one may address this question of future sex ratio, it certainly appears true that, as Helen Holmes concludes, the issue of sex selection 'forces us to confront sexism at its biological base and at the social level'.[12]

In the last resort, of course, should society feel, or come to feel, that widespread sex preselection is leading to an unhealthy social imbalance between the sexes, it will always be possible to influence individual choices by a variety of social means – by drawing public attention to what is happening and by giving a new dimension to responsible parenthood which takes into account the common good as well as the good of the individual family. Singer and Wells conclude that 'as a last resort couples might have to be taxed in accordance with the number of children they have of the preponderant sex'.[13] I find such a prospect morally distasteful because of its punitive tone, and because of the consequences which might follow – as, for instance, in China as a result of a similar social policy. But what else might society do if it decided that there was a need to remedy an imbalance of the sex ratio? In referring to the future possibility of the commercial marketing of self-administered methods of sex preselection, the Warnock report recommended that such products should be controlled by law in order to ensure that they were 'safe, efficacious and of an acceptable standard for use'.[14] And perhaps this precaution of legal product-control might suggest the further step of enacting legal measures to control their distribution, so limiting, or even at times prohibiting, their availability as a means of sex preselection. They might always remain available on medical prescription – to couples with a family history of sex-linked diseases for example. And perhaps other social criteria could be established to permit individual exceptions to a national policy of, for instance, discouraging too many boys in any particular generation. But, quite apart from the difficulties of applying such a restrictive policy, and of ensuring its observance, we must consider the guilt which might be wrongfully imputed to parents who happen to produce a child of the 'wrong' sex by natural means, and who felt they had to justify it. This leads to the wider objection, just as a punitive taxing system seems morally distasteful, that any suggestion of social engineering by prevention appears to have all the characteristics of being a major intrusion on the privacy and inherent freedom of couples to establish the family of their choice.

It appears, then, that if society is to exercise some influence on the sex preselection of children when this is considered necessary to correct a widespread imbalance of the sexes, it would have to be done by more positive means. And the objections raised against taxation or control do not appear to apply to society offering positive incentives, such as child allowances or attractive educational and other social opportunities, in order to encourage the birth of more girls, both for their future quality of life and for their public contributions to society; and possibly also to reverse a harmful decrease of future child-bearers in the total population.

In the light of all these considerations as we survey the ethics of the sex selection of children it may seem to some that we would do well not to open such a Pandora's box but leave things as they are, apart from the obvious medical benefits in some cases. To others it may appear that we are simply on the threshold of a further unavoidable stage in the biological and social development of our species, and this is the view which I tend in principle to favour. Widespread availability of a simple means of preselecting the sex of children will remove many ills from society by preventing the spread of sex-related diseases, eliminating the occasions for gender abortions, avoiding controversy over *in vitro* fertilisation, making some contribution to population-control, and even proving acceptable to those who oppose contraception. It will also respect the freedom of individuals and couples, increase their choices, and enable them to exercise responsible parenthood in the way which seems appropriate to them. And it will always allow for couples to choose not to avail themselves of it if they prefer to leave matters to nature or to a provident God, and for society to introduce compensating factors if and when such individual choices multiply to give rise to social concern.

As a final postscript, it may be worth observing that the sex selection of children for other than medical reasons may be thought only one step short of positive eugenics – that is, of taking steps not just to remedy deficiencies in the genetic constitution of humans but in some way to enhance them. One possible development against which the White Paper, *Human Fertilisation and Embryology*, has set its face is what it describes as one of the greatest causes of public disquiet about the newly developed techniques in human reproduction: the creation of human beings 'with certain predetermined characteristics through modification of an early embryo's genetic structure'.[15] And sex preselection undertaken in the positive interests of new human persons is perhaps not too far from genetic modification for the connection to be taken in all seriousness.

This consideration may invoke our old friend in such areas – the slippery slope. As an argument it is never one which I find compelling. For many of us spend a large part of our lives on slippery slopes. And, as one writer observed, when you are on a slippery slope, everything depends on whether you are wearing skis or crampons. In some cases when this argument is used it is really a rhetorical delaying tactic, intended to oppose action with a frightening red danger light. In other cases it may be a legitimate and salutary delaying argument, more of an amber light, and giving pause for thought. For it forces one to reflect and to give a clear explanation as to why it should be considered justifiable to go so far, without inevitably being dragged further than one had originally intended.

On the whole question of genetic modification, or (in this

case) of genetic preselection, there is fairly general agreement on its value for therapeutic purposes or for negative eugenics; and there is, thus, little concern about these possibilities. Where serious misgivings exist, they relate to attempts or desires, not to remedy or cure the genetic structure, but to improve or enhance it. The distinction between therapeutic and enhancing genetics is a useful clarification for practical ethical guidance, but it may have at least one potential ambiguity. It seeks to identify and make legitimate 'therapeutic' procedures which are aimed at curing or remedying conditions in individuals which fall short of the normal standard of health. But what would count as 'therapy' as our idea of health expands to include not only some desirable degree of physical, emotional and mental equilibrium but also some reasonable concern for social and environmental harmony and equilibrium? If that expansion of our understanding of health continues, may not the idea of desirable *remedial* or *therapeutic* genetic medicine expand into areas which have hitherto been judged to be undesirable *enhancing* genetic medicine and modification?

To pursue that speculation is not the purpose of this chapter. It may, nevertheless, prompt us to consider whether sex preselection is already a first tentative step in that general direction. If so, then the possible logical extension of such choices, for individuals as well as society, should serve to make us soberly aware that we are indeed moulding the lives of human individuals and possibly the contours of our future society. We should try, then, if not to stop at the red light, at least to proceed with the amber light with considerable caution and circumspection.

## Notes and references

1 Working Party of the Council for Science and Society. Human procreation. Oxford, Oxford University Press, 1984, paragraphs 1.8 and 5.9.

2 Department of Health and Social Security. Report of the Committee of Inquiry into Human Fertilisation and Embryology. Cmnd 9314 (Chairman: Dame Mary Warnock). London, HMSO, 1984, paragraphs 9.11–9.12.

3 Parliament. Human fertilisation and embryology: a framework for legislation. Cmnd 259. London, HMSO, 1987, pages 30 and 35.

4 See 2 above, paragraph 9.11.

5 R Steinbacher and Helen B Holmes. Sex choice: survival and sisterhood. In: C Gena and others (eds). Man-made women: how new reproductive technologies affect women. London, Hutchinson, 1985, page 60. Compare with Kevin T Kelly. Life and love. London, Collins, 1987, page 99.

6 Helen B Holmes and Betty B Hoskins. Prenatal and preconception sex choice technologies: a path to femicide? In: C Gena and others (eds). Man-made women: how new reproductive technologies affect women. London, Hutchinson, 1985, page 23.

7 Clifford Longley. Making the best of celibacy. The Times, 14 September 1987.

8 David Thomson. Europe since Napoleon. London, Longman, 1962, page 537.

9 M R Reinhard. Histoire de la population mondiale. Paris, page 580.

10 P Singer and D Wells. The reproductive revolution. Oxford, Oxford University Press, 1984, page 169.

11 See 8 above, page 538.

12 Helen B Holmes. Review of Gendercide: the implications of sex selection, by Mary Anne Warren. In: Bioethics, I, 1, 1987, page 104.

13 See 10 above, page 171.

14 See 2 above, paragraph 9.12.

15 See 3 above, page 37.

# Index

Aaron, H. 129
abortion
  argument against 11
  ethics 47–49, 145–6
  immorality of 69–72
  justification 62–67
  legislation on 47
  sex selection and 145–6
  women's rights and 65–67, 78
accountability of state in resource
  allocation 123–4
AIDS
  risk reduction 139
  tolerance towards 131–40
androgogy 86
Arendt, H. 130
Arrow, K.J. 129
autonomy, individual 17–18

Barnes, J. 77, 78
Barr, N. 129
Beske, F. 129
Black, D. 110–11, 115
Bosk, C.L. 112
British Medical Association views
  on euthanasia 15–33
  on fetal transplantation 48
Broad, C.D. 77
Brody, H. 93
Brown, J. 76
Bruer, J.T. 113
Brundage, D. 88
Byrne, P. 32, 76

California University Medical
  School 94, 95
Callah, S. et al. 129
Callahan, D.C. 105–6
Campbell, A.V. 88

Campbell, K. 77
Carter, S. 134
Chicago University Medical School
  94, 96–97, 102
Christianity
  attitude towards death and disease
  133–40
  sanctity of life and 38, 40–41
  see also religious
Clouser, K.D. 113, 114
consequential philosophy 20
consultation services on ethics
  99–100
Council for Science and Society 156
courses on ethics in USA 100–3
court decisions on euthanasia 4–5, 14
critical medical ethics 15
Culver, C.M. 114

Day, P. 130
death, attitude towards 133
DeCamp Conference 104–6
Department of Health
  responsibilities 125–6
Devine, P. 32
Devlin, H.B. 130
diagnosis, wrong, possibility of 13
disease
  attitude towards 133
  sex-related 145
doctors
  decision on euthanasia 5, 8, 12–13
  decision on medical treatment 3,
  19–24
  duties 18, 25
  morale 13
  options on abortion and fetal
  transplants 73–74
  relationship with patient 12, 18, 24

Downey, R.S. 88
drugs, costs vs benefits 126
Duncan, A.S. 112
Duncan, G.R. 112
Dunstan, G.R. 78
Dworkin, R.M. 78

Edwards, R. 141
Elkins, T. 101–2
embryo
  research 150
    ethics of 47–79
    immorality of 69–72
    justification 67–69
    use 49–53
European Convention for
    Protection of Human Rights
    and Fundamental Freedoms
    11
euthanasia
  active 4
  BMA's views on 15–33
  debate 10–13, 18
  definition 2–4
  for handicapped infants 24–29,
    38–40
  legislation decisions 4–6, 14
    proposals 6–9
  in Netherlands 1–14
  passive 4, 14
  role of courts 4–6
  unrequested 11–12
Evans, R.G. 129

Faden, R. *et al.* 32
fetal
  research, legislation on 59
  transplantation, ethics of 47–79
Finnis, J. 71, 78–79
*force majeure*, euthanasia and 5–6
freedom, State's role in 10–11

Gaita, R. 33
General Medical Council 112
Georgetown University 92
Gert, B. 114
Gilligan, C. 88
Gillon, R. 15, 88, 113
Goodman, N. 88

government *see* State
Green, F. 78
Greene, F. 46

Haksar, V. 78
handicapped
  infants, euthanasia for 24–29,
    38–40
  mentally, pregnancy and 81–82,
    83–85
Hare, R.M. 36
Hart, H. 34–35, 46
Hart, R.J. 114
Hartle, A. 109–10
Hastings Center 100, 113
Henderson, S.R. 114
Higgs, R. 88
hip replacements 116
HIV testing 139
Hogan, B. 32
Holmes, H.B. 157
homicide *see* 'killing'
homosexuals, attitude towards
    135–6
Hoskins, B.H. 157
Humanism, sanctity of life and
    40–41

*in vitro* fertilization, ethics of 141
infanticide
  acceptance of 39–40, 41
  historical view of 38
infants
  rights of 26–29, 55–57
  severely handicapped, euthanasia
    for 24–29, 38–40

Jameton, A.J. 113
Jonckheere, A.R. 79
Jonsen, A.R. 113

Kant, views on morals 49–62
Keele University 101
Kelly, K.T. 157
Kennedy, I. 33, 48–49, 58–59, 75, 76,
    79
Kennedy Institute of Medical Ethics
    100–1, 114
Kenny, A. 33

'killing'
distinction between 'letting die'
19–30
opportunistic 23–24
Society's views of 34–35
through omission 20–21
King's College 101
Klein, R. 130
Koop, E. 135
Kuhse, H. 32, 38–46

Leenan, H.J.J. 14
legislation
on abortion 47
on euthanasia 4–9, 14
on fetal research 59
on homicide 31–32
individual autonomy protection
and 17
leprosy, attitude towards 132
'letting die' distinction between
'killing' 19–30
life
mystery of 35–36
sanctity of 38–40
value of 34–36, 52
see also quality of life
Linacre Centre 32, 43, 46
Liverpool University 101
Lockwood, M. 76
Longley, C. 157

Mackeracher, D. 88
Macklin, R. 104
Magee, B. 87
Mahoney, Rev. J. 32, 35–36, 46
males, births after wars of 152
Manchester University 101
McElhinney, T.K. 113
McKellan, I. 140
medical education in USA 91
medical profession decision on
euthanasia 5
medical treatment
doctor's decision not to initiate or
terminate 3, 19–24, 43–45
new 13
process of dying and 10
refusal by patient 3–4

mentally handicapped, pregnancy
and 81–82, 83–85
Michigan University Medical School
93, 114
military ethics 109–10
mother's life, saving 61–64, 78–79

National Endowment for
Humanities 100
Nazis
euthanasia and 12
medical experiments by 75
neo-behaviourism 37
Netherlands, medical ethics in 1–14
Nolan, C. 133
non-consequential philosophy
20–21
Norman, R. 77
Nunn, J. 130

O'Neill, O. 87
organ transplants, ethics of 65–66

painkilling
aims of 3
techniques, euthanasia and 16
parental motives in sex selection
146–9
Parsons, J. 78
patient's decision on euthanasia 2–3,
7
competency of 12
Paton, H.J. 77
Pellegrino, E.D. 113, 114
Pennsylvania University Medical
School 92
Phillipp, E. 78
philosophy of euthanasia 20–21
Porter, R. & D. 32
Pratt, D.D. 88
pregnancy in mentally handicapped
81–82, 83–85

quality of life
deterioration in, euthanasia for 1,
21–22
evaluation 42–45
for handicapped infants 24–25,
30

Raphael, D.D. 77
Rawls, J. 130
Reich, W.T. 114
Reinhard, M.R. 157
relatives decision on euthanasia 9
religious attitude to sex selection
  143–4
  see also christianity; humanism
renal failure, end-stage 116
Rennie, D. et al. 129
resource allocation 116–30
right to life of infants 26–29, 55–57
Riker, W.H. 130
Ruddick, W. 104, 114

Schön, D.A. 83, 88
Schumpeter, J. 121, 130
Schwartz, W.B. 129
self-awareness 39–40
self-determination 2, 6, 10, 37, 42
Seller, M.J. 78
sex
  identification 142
  imbalance in society 149, 152–3
  selection 141–57
sexist attitudes to children 146–7,
  150–1
Siegler, M. 96–97, 108–9, 113
Singer, P. 38–46, 157
Skinner, B.F. 37, 46
Smith, J.C. 32
Somerville, M. 32
speciesism 38, 42
State
  Commission on Euthanasia in
    Netherlands 7–9, 14
  role in freedom 10–11
  role in resource allocation 117–30
Steinbacher, R. 157
Stone, J. 78
Stritch School of Medicine 93

teachers of medical ethics 108–9
  training 110–11
teaching medical ethics
  assessment and evaluation 107–8
  clinical 94–97

methods 111
objectives 103–7
in practice 80–88
postgraduate 97–103
practicalities 111–12
preclinical 92–94
premedical 91
in USA 89–115
Telfer, E. 88
Tennessee University Medical
  Center 101–2
termination of life see abortion;
  euthanasia
Texas University Medical Branch 92
Thomasma, D.C. 113
Thompson, J.J. 63–64, 78
Thomson, D. 157
tolerance in society 131–40
Tooley, M. 27–28, 33
Tucket, D. et al. 88

using people 51–56, 70–71

von Hügel, Baron 34
voting for resource allocation 120,
  121–3

Wales, University of 101
Ward, K. 76
Warnock Report, 76, 149–50, 156
Warren, M.A. 157
Warren, K.S. 113
Weale, A. 129
Weinfeld, J. 14
Welbourn, R.B. 112
Wells, D. 157
West Point Military Academy
  109–10
White, A.R. 33
will to live 35, 36
Williams, B. 33, 77
Williams, T. 135–6
wills, validity regarding euthanasia 3
Winslade, W.J. 113
women
  choice of sex in children 152
  rights, abortion and 65–67, 78